magpie / mm

MACROBIOTIC FOOD AND COOKING SERIES

Cooking for Health

ALLERGIES

by Aveline Kushi

edited by Rosalind Rhodes

foreword by Lawrence H. Kushi, Sc. D.

Japan Publications, Inc.

Tokyo • New York

Note to the reader: Those with health problems are advised to seek the guidance
of a qualified medical, or psychological professional in addition to qualified
macrobiotic counselor before implementing any of the dietary and other approaches presented in this book. It is essential that any reader who has any
reason to suspect serious illness in themselves or their family members seek
appropriate medical, nutritional, or psychological advice promptly. Neither this
or any other health related book should be used as a substitute for qualified
care or treatment.

Published by JAPAN PUBLICATIONS, INC., Tokyo and New York

Distributors:
UNITED STATES: *Kodansha International/USA, Ltd., through Harper & Row,
Publishers, Inc., 10 East 53rd Street, New York 10022.* SOUTH AMERICA:
Harper & Row, Publishers, Inc., International Department. CANADA: *Fitzhenry
& Whiteside Ltd., 195 Allstate Parkway, Markham, Ontario, L3R 4T8.* MEXICO
AND CENTRAL AMERICA: *HARLA S. A. de C. V., Apartado 30–546, Mexico 4,
D. F.* BRITISH ISLES: *International Book Distributors Ltd., 66 Wood Lane End,
Hemel Hempstead, Herts HP2 4RG.* EUROPEAN CONTINENT: *Fleetbooks, S. A.,
c/o Feffer and Simons (Nederland) B. V., Rijnkade 170, 1382 GT Weesp, The
Netherlands.* AUSTRALIA AND NEW ZEALAND: *Bookwise International, 1 Jeanes
Street, Beverley, South Australia 5007.* THE FAR EAST AND JAPAN: *Japan Publi-
cations Trading Co., Ltd., 1-2-1, Sarugaku-cho, Chiyoda-ku, Tokyo 101.*

First edition: May 1985
Second printing: January 1988

LCCC No. 84–081360
ISBN 0–87040–618–3

Printed in U.S.A.

Foreword ━━━━━━━━━━━━━━━━━━━━━━

The macrobiotic way of life is a common sense approach, based on tradition and reinforced by practice. It is most commonly identified as a diet that includes whole cereal grains, along with fresh vegetables, legumes and sea vegetables. It is becoming apparent that such a dietary pattern helps to prevent the development of chronic diseases, including most cardiovascular diseases and many cancers. It has also been suggested that such a dietary pattern may also diminish other health problems, such as allergies.

It is generally recognized that diet can affect the immune system, and therefore the underlying basis of allergic reactions, especially under severe circumstances. For example, several nutrients, including vitamins A and C, and iron and zinc can influence antibody response or lymphocyte function. Two of the most common causes of food allergies—eggs and milk— are not major components of a macrobiotic dietary pattern. Wheat, another cause of food allergy, can be and often is eaten less on a macrobiotic diet than on a typical Western diet

Many people report the diminishing or disappearance of symptoms of allergy after they have followed a macrobiotic diet. By incorporating the guidelines given in this book, and by putting the recipes into practice, you may experience similar benefits. On note, however: if you know that you have a hypersensitive reaction to some specific allergen, such as bee stings, penicillin or peanuts, please do not entertain the idea that the macrobiotic diet will eliminate these allergies. Macrobiotics can help you to develop a more common sense and holistic lifestyle, while improving the quality of your life, physical and otherwise.

LAWRENCE HARUO KUSHI, Sc. D.
February, 1985

Acknowledgments ▬▬▬▬▬▬▬▬▬▬

I would like to thank Japan Publications, Inc. for the opportunity to write this book and for their patience in waiting for the manuscript.

Thanks to Edward and Wendy Esko and Olivia Oredson for some preliminary research, outline and business arrangements.

Thanks to Rosalind Rhodes for co-writing the book.

Thanks to John D. Mann for overseeing the project, editing and contributing the chapter on *Understanding Allergies*.

Thanks to Onike Breedy for editing the chapter, *The Underlying Cosmology*. Thanks to Evelyne Harboun for proofreading and editing the recipes.

Thanks to Michio Kushi for writing the companion book, *Allergies (Macrobiotic Health Education Series)* as well as offering permission to use his notes on the *Standard Macrobiotic Diet* as well as some diagrams from his other books. Thanks to Mark Mead and John D. Mann for helping him write the book.

Thanks to Lily Kushi for the illustrations.

Also, thanks to Lawrence H. Kushi, Phillip Y. Kushi, Ann Rawley, Shigeko Ando, Mayumi Nishimura and Steve Gagne for extra comments and suggestions.

Contents

10

Introduction

About 20 years ago, after moving from New York City to Martha's Vineyard, I made a short return visit to Manhattan. While I was there I had dinner in a buffet style seafood restaurant and I tasted several kinds of fish as well as some boiled eggs.

After I went back to Martha's Vineyard, my whole neck started to itch and I started to scratch it. Then the skin of my neck became like snake skin or like fish scales. It was a very heavy rash. I knew the cause was the combination of fish and eggs, especially since I didn't eat these foods very often. I tried to adjust my food by completely eliminating all animal food. One day, two weeks later, I took a slice of lemon and I scrubbed lemon juice all over my neck. With a strong stinging sensation, surprisingly enough, the skin rash disappeared within minutes. I was really surprised. Two weeks of internal cleansing plus an external application worked to clear my neck. This is a very simple experience. This is my case.

I can't say this will definitely work for everyone. Each individual is different. Actually, everyday our skin condition changes. I am sure many people have noticed that some days there are pimples on the skin and some days there are spots, dark or red colors or patches. If you think about what you eat as you interact with the environment, you can notice how powerful food is and I can definitely say that with day to day food you can change your skin problems.

Limit animal food, sugar and chemicals. Watch your condition everyday. Look well at yourself in the mirror every morning. Check for flexibility in your body and your condition. When people eat macrobiotically for a while, their skin becomes more beautiful. We are always trying to improve the quality of our food. We just bought a small hulling machine for our rice so now we are able to retain the total vitality of the rice inside the hull up until the moment we cook it. I notice that our skin became much more beautiful as a result and we also feel more energetic. I invite you to try *macrobiotics*. There are no side-effects, it is economical and it doesn't harm our environment.

1. The Underlying Cosmology ━━━━━━━

There is a vast cosmology behind the principles of macrobiotics, a cosmology which sets out to explain the creation and the interrelationship of all phenomena throughout the universe to which we are a part.

The real purpose of macrobiotics is to empower us with the ability to fulfill our potentials and dreams and to serve as a reminder that we are the builders and masters of our own lives.

Macrobiotics is a rich and unlimited field of study that extends far beyond the scope of this book which you may feel free to pursue. In doing so, you will become your own guide, discovering for yourself what you need to do to maintain your health and to accomplish your personal goals. In this chapter is a brief overview of the underlying philosophy on which macrobiotics is based and how it applies to the aspects of diet and health.

Everything in the universe is a constantly moving and changing energy varying in density and speed. Even seemingly stable and solid objects, for instance, a rock or a table, are made up of moving molecules, atoms, electrons and protons which themselves are nothing but energy.

The origin and destination of all phenomena is Infinity, also called God, the Universal Will, the Super Consciousness or Nothingness. There is no time or space, past or future, light or darkness here. There is only endless motion, moving at an infinite speed in all directions.

These currents of endless motion (refer to Fig. 1) intersect and create logarithmic spirals which spin inwards towards the center in a contracting, centripetal (also referred to as the *yang* force) direction and opposite logarithmic spirals which spin outwards from the center in an expanding, centrifugal (also referred to as the *yin* force) direction. The formation of these spirals is how everything comes into being. In fact, these opposite but complimentary forces, by their constant interaction, are creating all things material and non-material. The Figure below shows the "Eternal and Universal Cycle of Change" reprinted from the *Book of Dō-In: Exercise for Physical and Spiritual Development* by Michio Kushi, (p. 18).

When moving in a yang (△) direction, the energy begins to take on more and more form in a process of materialization. Generally speaking, this process can be characterized by increasing speed, increasing temperature, and more density and weight which manifests as smallness or contraction, more material, hotter, faster, heavier and smaller. When moving in a yin (▽) direction energy takes on the opposite characteristics. It is less formed, more diffused, expanded, more cold, slower, and lighter. Yang

14

Fig. 1 The Eternal and Universal Cycle of Change.

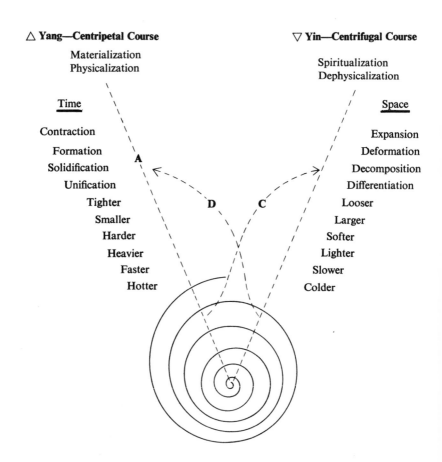

△ **Yang—Centripetal Course**

Materialization
Physicalization

<u>Time</u>

Contraction
Formation
Solidification
Unification
Tighter
Smaller
Harder
Heavier
Faster
Hotter

▽ **Yin—Centrifugal Course**

Spiritualization
Dephysicalization

<u>Space</u>

Expansion
Deformation
Decomposition
Differentiation
Looser
Larger
Softer
Lighter
Slower
Colder

A   D   C

motion is followed by yin, and yin motion is followed by yang. Yang does not exist without yin and vice versa.

All phenomena are created from these two opposite forces or directions of yin and yang which grew out of what we call God, Infinity, and so on. The spiral below is an illustration of the "Creation of the Universe." (Reprinted from the *Book of Dō-In: Exercise for Physical and Spiritual Development* by Michio Kushi, p. 23.)

Fig. 2   The Creation of the Universe.

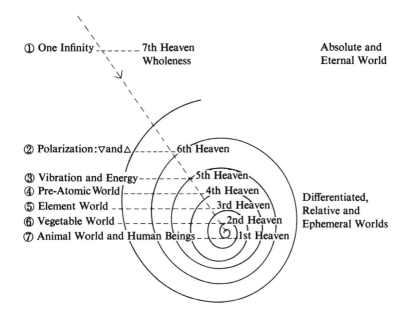

① One Infinity ⟍ _ _ _ _ _ 7th Heaven   Absolute and
                        Wholeness   Eternal World

② Polarization: ▽ and △ _ _ _ _ _ 6th Heaven
③ Vibration and Energy _ _ _ _ _ 5th Heaven
④ Pre-Atomic World _ _ _ _ _ _ _ _ 4th Heaven   Differentiated,
⑤ Element World _ _ _ _ _ _ _ _ _ 3rd Heaven   Relative and
⑥ Vegetable World _ _ _ _ _ _ _ _ 2nd Heaven   Ephemeral Worlds
⑦ Animal World and Human Beings _ _ _ 1st Heaven

① *One Infinity*:   Absolute and eternal, nothing but infinite motion.

② *Polarization—Yin (▽) and Yang (△)*:   The beginning of time and space, direction, dimensions, relativity, differentiation, and the ephemeral world.

③ *Vibration and Energy*:   The beginning of light, sound, long and short waves, the subconscious and conscious mind, mental and spiritual phenomena.

④ *Pre-Atomic World*:   The world of electrons, neutrons and other pre-atomic particles and the beginning of the material world.

⑤ *Element World*:   The world of molecules, the elements (hydrogen, helium, etc.), soil, water, air, fire, our senses and the beginning of the visible world.

⑥ *Vegetable World*:   The plant kingdom.

⑦ *Animal World and Human Beings*:   The animal kingdom including human beings.

Human beings, as the end result of a yang, centripetal spiral, are also at the beginning of a yin, centrifugal spiral. As we develop in a more yang direction we are created by physical food, the elemental energies from the sun, water, wind and so on, and the vibrations of thoughts from the mind. After we are formed in the physical world as we know it we start to go in the opposite yin direction as we develop emotionally, mentally and spiritually, and our body eventually decomposes and our soul later melts back into the infinite void.

The Figure below shows the "Eternal Cycle of Life." (Reprinted from the *Book of Dō-In: Exercise for Physical and Spiritual Development*. by Michio Kushi, p. 33.)

Fig. 3   The Eternal Cycle of Life.

Universal Will and Spirit
Infinite Speed of Motion

Universal Reincarnation

△ Physicalization Course   ▽ Spiritualization Course

Differentiation	Radiational Sphere	Spirit Life
Energization	Vibrational Sphere	Soul Life
Materialization	Plasmic Sphere	Astral and Ghost Life
Naturalization	Atmospheric Sphere	Human Life
Vegetalization	Water Sphere	Embryo and Fetus Life
Animalization	Mineral Sphere	Pre-embryonic Life

Conception
(Fusion)

Ovum
(Defusion)

Relative Speed of Motion
Finite Phenomenal World

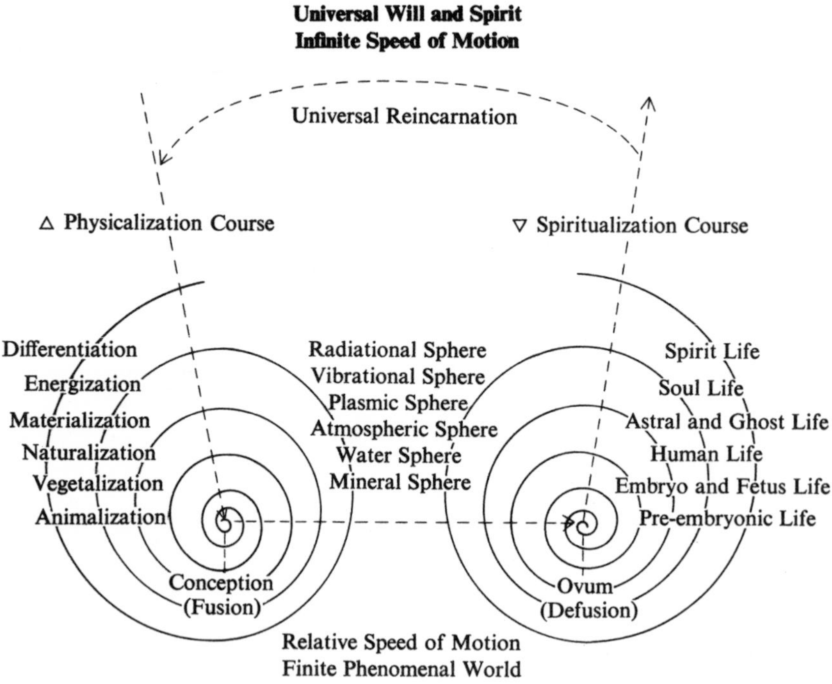

As you can see, the most contracted or yang point, the fusion of sperm and egg, is immediately followed by the yin, expanding force of rapid growth. (Yang in the extreme or at its peak turns into yin and vice versa.) This is followed by pre-embryonic life, which is followed by the watery and totally dark world of the embryo and fetus, followed by the airy atmosphere of our human environment as we know it. This world of air is half in darkness and half in light. When we pass away we shed our physical body and enter the plasmic astral world of ghosts or spiritual phenomena which is totally immersed in light. Each of the above successive worlds becomes more expansive, freer and involves a longer so-called time span.

By maintaining a healthy mind, body and spirit we are able to move more smoothly and happily into the next world. A pregnant woman has been traditionally told to get proper and balanced nourishment, sufficient exercise and rest, and to avoid violence in pastimes—movies, books and the like. She is also advised to send happy and beautiful thoughts to the baby so that the infant can come into this world in a healthy, happy state. In this way the child can live more peacefully and unencumbered. Likewise, in this life, we can all consider the quality of the various types of food we receive, the kinds of exercise and physical activity and rest we take, and encourage positive, creative thoughts and actions so that our birth into the next world will be smooth and our life there will be enjoyable. The spirits of unhappy persons are full of sorrow and delusion and instead of moving forward and onward into a brighter freer world of light, they remain attached to the earthly level and to the people and places they knew. The Oriental and other "primitive" cultures send their consolation, love, and wishes of happiness to their deceased ancestors. This helps to free these spirits and assists their ascent onto a broader and more joyful plane of existence.

We are all traveling back towards the outer parts of the universal spiral of life as we search for freedom, peace of mind, happiness, the ability to spread our wings and finally to be one with God. Even those who seemingly only want money or material possessions are actually looking for this same happiness and freedom and they feel it will result from their material pursuits. It is proper that each person pursues what he feels important at a given point. This is our freedom.

Paradoxically, we already are where we want to be as we ourselves are a miniature version of the whole universe at the same time that we are our small individual selves. Deep inside, each of us knows somehow that there is a larger I or self, a part of us which is eternal, all knowing and subject to no boundaries. There is a more synchronized feeling of unity, oneness and connection between our smaller I, our human existence, and our bigger I, this infinite universe, when we are in a relaxed, healthy, vibrant, in tune with nature state. We can tap into the unlimited, creative potential that we have in the universe and use it to direct our life with much more awareness when we are in harmonious synchronicity.

The deeper meaning of health is being in this aligned and synchronous state which results in a smooth, unblocked, effortless flow of our energies between all the inner and outer universal parts of ourselves. The macrobiotic approach to well-being is a holistic approach directed by our understanding that a change in any aspect or portion of our body or self has an effect on everything else including the world and the universe. There are several approaches one can take to create a free flow of energy:

1. *Changing your diet:* This is the perspective that this book basically focuses on. What we eat creates our blood cells, and hence the formation of our organs and all other parts of our body. It is a wonder that food is not often associated as a major cause of disease. One's diet also alters the mind and emotions. We know that the ingestion of alcohol and various licit and illicit drugs effects one's mental state. This fact cannot be argued. Likewise, anything else one takes in has its effect on our being, though it may be on a subtle level.

2. *Working with the powers of the mind:* Everything that exists has its origin in the invisible world of the mind and vibrations. It is said that what we believe manifests. There are many negative thoughts or assumptions that we may dwell on which can influence our lives. Many of these delusions, as we may call them here, occur automatically and unconsciously. One may develop self-awareness by constantly observing the thoughts, actions, and reactions that control one's life and rechannel unwanted habits into more positive ideas and dreams.

3. *Relaxation:* Mental and physical tension block the freest flow of energy. A technique one may try is to take an inventory of all the parts of your body and relax all tense spots. You can do the same thing with the mind, letting go of anxiety, guilt and anger. Use the breath to help the relaxation process: breathe slowly and deeply.

4. *Palm-healing, shiatsu massage, moxibustion, acupuncture and chiropractics:* These practices can be used to temporarily unblock stagnations of energy in the body.

5. *Keep mentally and physically active:* Exercise, do sports or dancing, clean your house, garden, read, study, engage in hobbies, draw, write,

compose, play music, do volunteer work, teach . . . whatever you want. Make sure to do both mental and physical work. The more energy we circulate, the more comes back to us and the less stagnation there is in our lives.

6. *Changing ones environmental surroundings:* In some cases, it might be necessary to change ones environmental surroundings. Some forms of sicknesses can be more easily eliminated in a warm climate while others may require cooler temperatures. Moving to a quieter locale, like the countryside may be beneficial for some conditions. Also, it's important that one be in a loving atmosphere with people who care about you and give you support. Also, one can help to maintain a clean, unpolluted, ecologically balanced world by using biodegradable materials as much as possible, not taking more than one needs, as well as helping to protect the well-being of our fellow inhabitants on this earth—the members of the plant and animal kingdoms.

7. *Maintain good relationships with all the people in your life:* Blaming, holding grudges, anger, fear and hatred makes one very tense and causes blockages. We create the circumstances of our individual lives so it is up to us to change them. Give everyone your love, support, and respect for their freedom and individuality.

8. *Be grateful and thankful for all that you have been given:* Notice all the beauty and marvels in the world. Look at any hardships, difficulties, or rejections you encounter as opportunities for self-reflection and growth.

Working on just one of the above recommendations can be tremendously helpful and have a positive effect on us overall but to make a really permanent and thorough change for the better, all of the above should be worked on as they are interrelated. Many people form an exclusive allegiance to one approach and as time passes they wonder why their plans and dreams don't progress beyond a certain point. They then abandon their one approach and either give up or make an exclusive attachment to another approach. Please beware of this tendency.

Yin and Yang

Everything is created and governed by the interactions of yin and yang, the two opposite poles which are endlessly manifesting in the world. Below is a chart of some classification examples:

Attribute	Yin/Centrifugal (▽)	Yang/Centripetal (△)
Tendency	Expansion	Contraction
Function	Dispersion, decomposition	Assimilation, organization
Movement	More inactive, slower	More active, faster
Vibration	Shorter waves, high frequency	Longer waves, low frequency
Direction	Vertical; ascending	Horizontal, descending
Position	More outward and peripheral	More inward and central
Weight	Lighter	Heavier
Temperature	Colder	Hotter
Light	Darker	Lighter
Humidity	More wet	More dry
Density	Thinner	Thicker
Size	Larger	Smaller
Shape	More expanded, fragile	More contracted, harder
Length	Longer	Shorter
Texture	Softer	Harder
Atomic particle	Electron	Proton
Elements	N, O, K, P, Ca	H, C, Na, As, Mg
Environment	Vibration→Air→Water→	Earth
Climate	Tropical	Arctic
Biological	Vegetable	Animal
Sex	Female	Male
Organ structure	Hollow, expansive	Compact, condensed
Nerves	Orthosympathetic	Parasympathetic
Attitude	Gentle, negative	Active, positve
Work	Psychological & mental	Physical & social
Consciousness	More universal	More specific
Mental function	Dealing with the future	Dealing with the past
Culture	Spiritually oriented	Materially oriented
Color	Purple→Blue→Green→Yellow→	Brown→Orange→Red
Season	Winter	Summer
Dimension	Space	Time
Taste	Hot→sour→sweet→	Salty→Bitter
Vitamins	C	K, D
Catalyst	Water	Fire

By learning how yin and yang relate to each other you can begin to understand all the workings of the world. *I-Ching, The Book of Changes,* is based on yin-yang interactions. Macrobiotic dietary principles are drawn from this base.

Yin attracts yang and yang attracts yin, resulting in the harmony and marriage of two opposites. Examples are; man and woman, plus and minus magnets or electrical charges, electron and proton, spirit and matter, and so on. Upon injesting a quantity of salt (yang) for instance, one is then attracted to liquids (yin).

Yin repels yin, yang repels yang. Examples are: oil and water (both yin) don't mix. Two plus poles repel each other as do two minus poles.

The force of attraction (or repulsion as the case may be) is proportional to the ratio of the yin and yang elements. Their combination in various proportions creates an infinite variety of energies and phenomena where no two things in existence are identical.

Yin and yang are not static and are always flowing from one to another in various degrees. Yin in the extreme changes to yang and vice versa. Nothing lasts forever. Day turns into night, night into day. Activity is followed by rest, rest by activity. Success follows failure and failure follows success. Civilizations rise and fall. What has a beginning has an end.

Nothing is totally yin or totally yang. All things are made up of both. The more yin something is, the more yang it is as well. Many people that appear yang, strong, rough and tough on the outside may in comparison be yin, weak, and fragile on the inside. Others that appear yin, soft, and fragile on the outside may well be yang, strong and stubborn on the inside. Something that is structurally yang, as is the dense and compacted liver, is energetically yin; it functions without much motion. Things that are structurally yin, as a hollow heart, are energetically more yang, as it never stops pumping, contracting and expanding. The bigger the front, the bigger the back.

Large yin attracts small yin, large yang attracts small yang. After you take sugar (large yin) you are drawn to drinking more fluids (small yin).

Yin creates yang, yang creates yin. A yin, colder climate creates yang, small, hardy vegetation and a more yang, ambitious, hard-driving society. While a yang, warmer climate creates yin, watery, large, lush vegetation and a more slow paced, easy going and relaxed society.

Everything on this earth is created by varying proportions of upward and downward energies. Gravity is an example of downward energy. The growth of trees and plants is an example of upward energy.

Yin and Yang and Diet —————————————————————————————

Yang foods give warmth, strength, discipline and vitality. Excessively yang foods (such as red meat, eggs or too much salt) are known to cause rigidity, egocentricity, exclusivity, constrictions, restlessness, arthritic conditions, heart attacks, violent tendencies and the like.

Yin foods are cooling, cleansing, relaxing and nurture patience and understanding. Excessively yin foods (such as honey, sugar, chemicals and drugs) have been shown to cause weakening and dispersion of the functioning capabilities in body and mind, including fear, defensiveness, loss of will, suspectibility to so-called viruses, a rampage of white blood cell production, and depression or suicidal tendencies, to name some common problems.

When taking in overly yang foods, one is automatically attracted to overly yin ones (and vice versa) to make balance and compensation. One may end up on a wild or chaotic seesaw with a combination of unwanted side-effects such as the ones listed above. Macrobiotics recommends a diet of more centrally balanced foods. Grains are the most centered and appropriate foods for human beings, requiring only a minimum amount of counterbalancing. (Grains are our complementary opposites as they are the last stage of plant evolution just as we are the last stage of animal evolution.) Brown rice, especially, has the right proportions of yin and yang for humans and provides the most stabilizing dietary staple.

Humans are constitutionally yang, warm-blooded beings and therefore require most if not all of their nourishment from their complementary opposite, which is the yin, vegetable kingdom. Among animal foods, fish is the recommended choice, particularly slow moving, white-meat varieties as well as some shellfish. The human digestive system doesn't digest or assimilate meat well. It lingers and putrefies in the stomach. The only circumstance where it is healthy to eat large amounts of animal food is in the very cold, yin, arctic regions where more strongly yang food is needed and where the availability of plant food is minimal.

Actually, climate plays a major role in our choice of available edibles. It is recommended that we choose fresh produce which is grown or can grow in our own climatic zone. Tropical fruits are more appropriate when consumed where they are grown but they are detrimental to one's health when taken in large quantities or too regularly in the temperate zone.

The seasons as well play an important part in food selection. For instance, in the spring when the energy is rising and expanding we should include fresh young greens and sprouts. Towards fall and then winter, when the energies are descending and contracting, squash, kale, and winter

Fig. 4   General Yin (▽) and Yang (△) Categorization of Food.

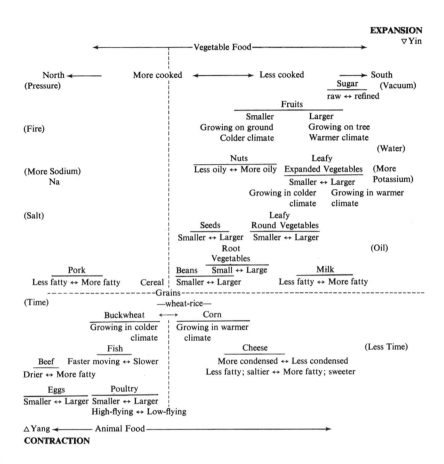

The above chart gives the general idea of the classification of food groups from yang to yin, from yin to yang. However, more precise classification should be made upon examination of environmental conditions, nature and structure, chemical compounds, and effect upon our physical and mental conditions. Also, cooking can greatly change food qualities from yin to yang and yang to yin.

storable vegetables such as root vegetables, and dried plants such as sea vegetables should be consumed.

A variety of cooking methods should be employed as well. In the winter, we can eat more well-cooked, slightly saltier, pressure-cooked, and baked foods as well as more fish. In the summer more lightly-cooked, boiled, raw (such as salads and fruit), chilled and steamed foods and desserts may be consumed.

Also, within one meal we should ideally have a representation of a variety of cooking styles as well as a variety of tastes, color and sizes.

Two additional factors which determine what is yin and what is yang and to what relative degree are: (1) rate of growth (faster is more yin and slower is more yang) and (2) portion of the plant being considered— whether roots (more yang) or leaves and fruits (more yin), and so on.

The preceding chart, from the *Book of Macrobiotics: The Universal Way of Health and Happiness* by Michio Kushi, p. 57, represents a general yin/yang categorization of foods.

2. Explanation of the Standard Macrobiotic Diet —————

These dietary recommendations are suggested for individuals in a general sound state of health. Persons having a more serious condition may need further modifications. It should also be noted that this is a general guideline and no matter what your condition, each person's individuality, lifestyle and environment need to be taken into account with the diet adapted accordingly.

To see exactly what foods are recommended, refer to the detailed food list following the section below on proportions.

1. WHOLE CEREAL GRAINS. It is recommended that at least 50% of every meal include cooked, organically grown, whole cereal grains prepared in a variety of ways.

2. SOUPS. Approximately 5–10% of your daily food intake (one or two bowls daily) may include soup made with traditional and naturally processed *miso* or *tamari* soy sauce. The flavor should not be overly salty, and your soup may include a variety of grains, beans and vegetables, including sea vegetables such as *wakame* and *kombu*.

3. VEGETABLES. About 20–30% of each meal may include local and organically grown vegetables with a large amount cooked in various styles and a smaller amount eaten as raw salad.

4. BEANS AND SEA VEGETABLES. Approximately 5–10% of your daily diet may include cooked beans and sea vegetables.
    Sea vegetables may be prepared in a variety of ways. They can be cooked with beans or vegetables, used in soups, or cooked and eaten separately as side dishes, flavored with a moderate amount of *tamari* soy sauce, sea salt, or rice vinegar.

5. SUPPLEMENTARY FOODS. Approximately 5–10%. Once or twice weekly a small amount of fresh white-meat fish may be eaten if desired.
    Fruit desserts, including fresh and dried fruits, may also be consumed on occasion. Local and organically grown fruits are preferred. Frequent use of fruit juice is not advisable. However, occasional con-

sumption in warmer weather is allowable, depending on your health.

Lightly roasted seeds may be enjoyed as a snack. Though less frequently, some roasted nuts may be consumed. Rice syrup and barley malt may be used occasionally to add a sweet taste; rice vinegar or *umeboshi* vinegar may also be used occasionally for a sour taste.

6. BEVERAGES. Any traditional tea which does not have an aromatic fragrance or a stimulant effect can be used such as *bancha* (*kukicha*) twig tea, and roasted grain teas. You may also drink a moderate amount of water (preferably spring or well water). Iced drinks are best avoided.

7. FOODS TO BE AVOIDED FOR BETTER HEALTH. Meat, eggs, animal fat, poultry, dairy products, including butter, yogurt, ice cream, milk and cheese.

Tropical or semi-tropical fruits and fruit juices, soda, artificial drinks and beverages, coffee, colored tea, and all aromatic, stimulant teas such as mint and peppermint tea.

All artificially colored, preserved, sprayed, or chemically treated foods. All refined polished grains, flours and their derivatives. Mass-produced industrialized food including all canned and frozen foods.

Hot spices, any aromatic, stimulant food or food accessory; artificial vinegar and other seasonings. Licit and illicit drugs are best avoided. (Medicines prescribed by a physician do not apply to this general guideline.) Alcohol and cigarettes should be kept to a minimum.

8. ADDITIONAL SUGGESTIONS. Cooking oil should be vegetable quality only. If you wish to improve your health use only cold-pressed mechanically expelled unrefined sesame or corn oil in moderate amounts.

Salt should be naturally processed sea salt and excessive use should be avoided. Traditional, non-chemicalized *tamari* or *shoyu* sauce and *miso* may also be used like sea salt.

You may eat regularly two to three times per day, as much as you want, provided the proportion is correct and chewing is thorough (at least 50 times per mouthful or until it becomes liquid). Please avoid eating for approximately three hours before sleeping.

A More Detailed Macrobiotic Food List ———————

Items marked with an asterisk (*) are foods that may have to be avoided or restricted when trying to cure some illnesses; look under the list of diet modifications for specific diseases for more information.

Grains: ——————————————————————————

Regular use	Occasional use	Occasional flour products
Short grain brown rice	Long grain brown rice	Whole wheat noodles*
Medium grain brown rice	Sweet brown rice	Udon noodles*
	Mochi	Somen noodles*
Barley	Cracked wheat, bulghur	Soba noodles (buckwheat)*
Pearl barley	Steel cut oats	
Millet	Rolled oats*	Unyeasted whole wheat bread*
Corn	Corn grits*	
Corn on the cob	Corn meal*	Unyeasted rye bread*
Whole oats	Rye Flakes	Fu*
Whole wheat berries	Couscous	Seitan*
Buckwheat*		
Rye		

Vegetables: ——————————————————————

Regular use	Occasional use	Avoid
Acorn squash	Celery*	Artichoke
Bok choy	Chives*	Bamboo shoots
Broccoli	Coltsfoot*	Beets
Brussels sprouts	Cucumber*	Curley dock
Burdock	Endive*	Eggplant
Butternut squash	Escarole*	Fennel
Cabbage	Green beans*	Ferns
Carrots & their tops	Green peas*	Ginseng
Cauliflower	Iceberg lettuce*	Green & red peppers
Chinese cabbage	Jerusalem artichoke*	New Zealand spinach
Collard greens	Kohlrabi*	Okra
Daikon & their tops	Lambsquarters*	Plantain
Dandelion roots, leaves	Mushrooms*	Purslane & sheperd's purse
Hubbard squash	Patty-pan squash*	
Hokkaido pumpkin	Romaine lettuce*	Potato
Jinenjo	Salsify*	Sorrel
Kale	Shiitake mushrooms*	Spinach
Leeks	Snap beans*	Sweet potato
Lotus root	Snow peas*	Swiss chard

Mustard greens
Onion
Parsley
Parsnip
Pumpkin
Radish
Red cabbage
Rutabaga
Scallions
Turnips & greens
Watercress

Sprouts*
Summer squash*
Wax beans*

Tomato
Taro potato (albi)
Yams
Zucchini

Beans:

Regular use	Occasional use	Occasional bean substitutes
Azuki beans	Black-eyed peas*	Dried *tofu*
Black soybeans	Black turtle beans*	Fresh *tofu**
Chickpeas (garbanzos)	Great northern beans*	*Natto**
Lentils (green)	Kidney beans*	*Tempeh**
	Lima beans*	
	Mung Beans*	
	Navy beans*	
	Pinto beans*	
	Soybeans*	
	Split peas*	
	Whole dried peas*	

Sea Vegetables:

All these sea vegetables can be used regularly. *Arame, Hijiki, Kombu,* toasted *Nori, Wakame,* Dulse, Agar-agar, Irish moss, *Mekabu.*

Fruits (usually cooked or dried):

Occasional use	Avoid
Apples*	Avocados
Apricots*	Bananas
Blueberries*	Coconuts
Blackberries*	Dates
Cantaloupes*	Figs
Cherries*	Grapefruit
Grapes*	Kiwi fruit
Lemons (small amounts of juice for cooking)*	Oranges
	Mangoes
Peaches*	Papayas

Pears*
Plums*
Raisins*
Raspberries*
Strawberries*
Watarmelon*

Persimmons
Pineapple
All other tropical fruits

Seeds and Nuts:

Occasional use
Almonds*
Chestnuts*
Peanuts*
Pumpkin seeds*
Sesame seeds*
Sunflower seeds*
Walnuts*

Avoid
Brazil nuts
Caraway seeds
Cashews
Hazel nuts
Macadamian nuts
Pistachios
Poppy seeds
Spanish peanuts
All tropical nuts

Animal Foods and Their Products:

Occasional use
Carp*
Clams*
Cod*
Flounder*
Halibut*
Lobster*
Oysters*
Trout*
Red snapper*
Sole*
White-meat fish in general*

Avoid
Red-meat fish
Chicken
All fowl
Eggs
All mammals
All dairy products

Pickles:

Regular use
Bran pickles
Brine pickles
Miso bran pickles
Miso pickles
Pressed pickles
Sauerkraut
Tamari Pickles
Takuan Pickles

Avoid
Commercial dill pickles
Herb pickles
Garlic pickles
Spiced pickles
Apple cider vinegar pickles
Wine vinegar pickles

Sweets:

Regular use	Occasional use	Avoid
Cabbage	Amazake*	All tropical fruits
Carrots	Barley malt*	Brown sugar
Daikon	Chestnuts*	Carob
Onions	See fruit list*	Chocolate
Parsnips	Hot apple cider*	Fructose
Pumpkin	Hot apple juice*	Honey
Squash	Rice malt syrup*	Maple syrup
		Molasses
		White sugar

Beverages:

Regular use	Occasional use	Infrequent use	Avoid
Bancha twig tea (Kukicha)	Grain coffee (100% grain)	Green tea*	Distilled water
Bancha stem tea	Dandelion tea	Vebetable juices*	Coffee
Roasted barley tea	Kombu tea	Juices of fruits from fruit list*	Cold, iced drinks
Roasted brown rice tea	Umeboshi tea	Beer*	Hard liquor
Spring water	Mu tea	Saké*	Herb teas
Well water			Mineral water & all bubbly water
			Regular tea
			Stimulants
			Sugared drinks
			Tap water
			Whisky
			Wine

Seasonings and Oils:

Regular use	Occasional use	Avoid
Natural miso	Corn oil*	Animal fats
Dark sesame oil*	Ginger*	Butter & cream
Light sesame oil*	Horseradish*	Coconut oil
Natural soy sauce	Mirin*	Cottonseed oil
Tamari soy sauce	Olive oil*	Commercial dressings
Unrefined white sea salt	Rice vinegar*	Garlic
Umeboshi plum & paste	Safflower oil*	Linseed oil
Umeboshi vinegar	Sunflower oil*	Margarine
		Mayonnaise
		Commercial miso
		Mustard
		Pepper

Peanut oil
Table salt
All commercial season-
ings
Soybean oil
Commercial soy sauce
All spices

Condiments:

Main condiments	Other condiments
Gomashio (sesame salt)	Brown rice vinegar
Sea vegetable powder	Cooked miso with scallions &
Sea vegetable powder with roasted	onions
sesame seeds	Nori condiment
Tekka	Roasted sesame seeds
Umeboshi plum	Shiso leaves & roasted sesame seeds
	Shio Kombu
	Umeboshi plum with raw scallions/
	onions
	Umeboshi vinegar

Snacks:

You can have leftovers, noodles, popcorn (unbuttered), puffed whole cereal grain, rice balls, rice cakes, roasted seeds, sushi, and whole wheat bread.

Cooking and Preparation Methods:

Regular use	Occasional use
Pressure cooking	Sautéing*
Boiling	Stir-frying*
Steaming	Raw*
Waterless	Deep-frying*
Soup	Tempura*
Pickling	Baking*
Oilless sautéing (with water)	
Pressing	

Cooking Aspects to Change for Variety:

1. Selection of foods within the categories of grains, vegetables, beans, sea vegetables, and so on;
2. Methods of cooking;
3. Ways of cutting vegetables;
4. Amount of water used;
5. Amount and kind of seasoning and condiments used;

6. Length of cooking time;
7. Use of a higher or lower flame;
8. Varying the combination of foods and dishes;
9. Seasonal cooking adjustments.

Way of Life Suggestions and Reminders ──────────

- Maintain the dream and image of health, peace, and abundance for yourself, others and the world.
- Live each day happily without being preoccupied with your health, stay mentally and physically alert and active.
- View everything and everyone you meet with gratitude. Offer thanks before and after each meal.
- It is best to retire before midnight and get up early in the morning, especially with the sunrise.
- It is best to avoid wearing synthetic or woolen clothing directly against the skin. Wear cotton as much as possible, especially for undergarments. Avoid excessive metallic accessories on the fingers, wrists, or neck. Keep such ornaments simple and graceful.
- If your strength permits, go outdoors in simple clothing. Walk on the grass, beach, or soil up to one half hour every day.
- Keep you home (and other surroundings) in good order, from the kitchen, bathroom, bedroom, living room, to every corner of the house.
- Initiate and maintain an active correspondence, extending best wishes to your family and friends. Also maintain and initiate good relationships with everyone around you.
- Avoid taking long hot baths or showers unless you have been consuming too much salt or animal food.
- Scrub your entire body with a hot, damp towel until the skin becomes red, every morning or every night before retiring. If that is not possible, at least scrub your hands, feet, fingers and toes.
- Avoid chemically-perfumed cosmetics. For care of the teeth, brush with natural preparations or sea salt.
- If your condition permits, exercise regularly as part of your daily life, including activities like scrubbing floors, cleaning windows and so on as well as exercise programs such as yoga, dance, sports, and martial arts.
- Avoid using electric cooking devices (ovens or ranges) or microwave ovens. Convert to a gas or wood stove at the earliest opportunity.
- It is best to minimize the frequent use of color television and computer display units.
- Include some large green plants in your house to freshen and enrich the oxygen content of the air in your home.

3. Dietary Adjustment for Allergies ▬▬▬

So far, we have looked at the *Standard Macrobiotic Diet*. To relieve an allergic condition it is necessary to initially adjust this diet further for some period of time, usually about two to three months, until the condition begins to improve.

To be allergic in the first place, one's blood quality and immune system have to already be in a weak state. We try to understand why some people are allergic and others are not, and instead of avoiding the external triggers, we deal with the original, underlying cause within ourselves.

I strongly recommend that you read the companion book *Allergies* by Michio Kushi, published by the same publisher as this book. This will help you to gain an understanding of the working of allergies and therefore assist you to relieve the conditions in a more conscious and aware manner.

An excessive intake of the following foods contributes to one's susceptibility; dairy products, oil and grease (especially animal fats), refined flour, fruits and their juices (especially tropical fruits), poultry and eggs (especially in the case of skin allergies), sugar, honey, soft drinks, fish (especially blue-skin fish, particularly for skin allergies), raw foods, spices, drugs and chemicals.

Listed below are some general suggestions for allergies:

1. Minimize oatmeal, flakes and grits. Avoid baked flour products, especially those with yeast. If you crave bread, have some natural sourdough or unleavened bread on occasion. Stay away from pies, cakes and pastries for now.
2. Have *miso* soup or *miso* rice everyday.
3. Limit or avoid "occasional use" vegetables, emphasizing those for "regular daily use." Avoid raw foods in the beginning except pickles. You may make quickly boiled or pressed salad instead.
4. Minimize your intake of oil, using it only for lightly sautéed vegetables once or twice a week, if you really desire it. Use dark sesame oil.
5. Initially reduce your intake of beans and bean products, using smaller portions of the "regular use" beans (*azuki*, lentil and chickpeas) only. Among bean products, dried *tofu* is the best to use.
6. Be especially light on all salt seasonings including *tamari* soy sauce, *miso* and *umeboshi*.
7. Generally avoid nuts and nut or seed butters. Roasted seeds are alright to use.

8. It's best to stay away from fruit initially. If you crave it, eat a little bit of cooked, dried fruit taken from the "recommended" fruit list in the standard recommendations, once or twice a week. If you crave a sweet taste in general, first try satisfying it by eating sweet vegetables such as squash, carrots, onions, parsnips, etc. Further, you can prepare delicious desserts using grain-based sweeteners, chestnuts, and other non-fruit ingredients. Then, if you still crave an even sweeter taste, eat the fruit.

9. Minimize animal food, take only white-meat fish, once or twice a week at the most and only if you truly desire it.

10. No spices (including mustard, pepper, and curry).

11. Make sure to include both lightly-cooked and well-cooked foods daily.

12. Good digestion is very important so it is imperative to chew very well.

13. Pay particular attention to vigorously scrub your body with a hot, damp towel once a day for good circulation.

• *Additional advice for specific allergies:*

Hay Fever

Possible symptoms: A runny nose, watery and itchy eyes, fever, ear pain, fatigue, irritability, moodiness and headaches.

Possible triggers: Pollen from grass, plants and trees, especially during the spring and summer months. The same people can also be allergic to house dust, mold and animal fur.

1. Often use lotus root (fresh or dried) or lotus seeds in cooking. Other hardy root vegetables (burdock, *daikon*, dandelion, etc.) also help to strengthen the lungs and respiratory system.

2. Reduce the volume of beans and bean products.

3. It is best to refrain from any oil for one to two months. Avoid nuts, and nut and seed butters.

4. Take a half a cup of lotus root juice for five days and then twice a week. Heat it with a pinch of sea salt.

5. If you get constipated, take agar-agar with rice or barley malt.

6. Apply a lotus root plaster on the forehead and sinus area, around the eye. (You can sleep with it overnight.) More than one application may be needed.

7. Avoid dusty places. Try to surround yourself with clean air.

Asthma ──────────────────────────

Possible symptoms: Attacks of extreme breathing difficulties and wheezing, coughing, and heavy mucus.

Possible triggers: There is much speculation here. Triggers have seemed to include dust, pollen, animal fur, foods, respiratory tract infection, aspirin, plastic fumes, chemical dusts (*platinum*) and gases (*toluene*) as well as other chemicals and the spores of *Aspergillus fumigatus*.

1. Cook regularly with a lot of lotus root (fresh or dried) and lotus seeds, mixing them in with grains and vegetables.
2. Take special care to use a small volume of condiments, especially fresh *gomashio* and *umeboshi*, everyday.
3. Avoid salad and fruits and their juices.
4. Avoid excessive liquids and all cold beverages. Use the drinks in the *Special Needs* chapter to speed relief.
5. If you get constipated, take agar-agar with rice or barley malt.
6. If you have a coughing attack you may take:
    A. 1 cup hot *bancha* tea with 1 tablespoon barley malt or
    B. 1 bowl of *kuzu* with 1 tablespoon barley malt or
    C. 1–2 cups of hot *amazake* with optional *kuzu*.
7. Apply a mustard plaster or ginger compress on your back and chest several times a week, to help dissolve stagnated mucus and fat.
8. Avoid wet, damp surroundings.

Skin Allergies (including Hives, Angioedema, Eczema) ─

Possible Symptoms: *Hives*—Itchy skin, pale and raised bumps of varying sizes which are often surrounded by an area of redness and warmth. *Angioedema*—Swelling of the lips, tongue, eyelids, throat, sex organs and mucus membranes. *Eczema*—Itchy, red, dry skin.

Possible triggers: There is much speculation here also. Triggers have seemed to be foods (particularly eggs, shellfish, nuts or fruits), a variety of medications, chemicals, pollens, insect stings, sunlight, cold temperatures, infections, parasites, exercise and certain illnesses of adjustment.

1. Avoid buckwheat and its flour, including *soba* noodles.
2. Have *nishime* vegetables daily or every other day for one month (particularly *daikon* with its leaves and *kombu*, adding a little *tamari* soy sauce or *miso* to taste).

3. Reduce the volume of beans and their products.
4. Avoid salad and fruit.
5. Avoid fish. If you strongly crave it, have a small portion of white-meat fish mixed in with vegetables. Strictly avoid red-meat and blue-skin fish, and shellfish.
6. Avoid sunflower seeds as well as nuts. Roasted sesame and pumpkin seeds are OK.
7. Take a cup of *azuki* bean juice daily for five to seven days and then twice a week. Add a pinch of sea salt.
8. If your skin is inflamed or irritated, make either one of these two plasters:
   A. A rice bran plaster with green leafy vegetables or
   B. A green *nori* plaster with green leafy vegetables
9. Wear 100 percent cotton, especially against the skin.
10. Scrub your body with a rice-bran wash (see *Special Needs* chapter).

Food Allergies

Possible symptoms: Eczema, hives, diarrhea, vomiting, cramps, nasal irritation and discharge, indigestion.

Possible triggers: Various foods including dairy products, eggs, wheat products, corn products, chocolate, nuts, fruits, mustard, legumes, tomatoes, sweets, seafood (especially shellfish), and various meats.

Tests for food allergies may not always be accurate as different combinations with other foods, different cooking styles and the amount of chewing can vary the items greatly. Allergies to foods which are not included in the *Standard Macrobiotic Diet*, are actually the body's natural reaction to harmful substances. This is particularly true for dairy products.

1. Avoid the food to which you are allergic. After three months, have some (if the particular item is a part of standard macrobiotic eating) and see if the allergy still persists. If it does, continue following the recommendations for a while longer.
2. Make sure to have some *miso* soup and a small amount of sea vegetables everyday.
3. Items to be taken daily or every other day for one month:
   A. 1 cup *kombu* juice (boiled down from two cups of water)
   B. ½–1 of an *umeboshi* plum or the equivalent amount of *shiso* leaves in *bancha* tea or as a condiment with rice or other grains.

C. Some kind of sea vegetable condiment such as *shio-kombu,* roasted *wakame* or *nori* condiment.
4. Chewing well is particularly important, at least 50 times a mouthful.

Chemical Allergies

Possible symptoms: Some of the above allergies; and if left unchecked, they can further develop into cancer, arthritis, cataracts, atherosclerosis, impotence and sterility.

Possible triggers: Chemical additives in foods, toxic fumes, factory smoke, aerosol sprays, automobile exhaust, and other pollutions around us.

1. Pay careful attention to getting as much organic food as possible.
2. Eat *nishime* vegetables two to three times a week for two to three months.
3. Have brown rice, *miso* soup and sea vegetables everyday. *Miso* rice can be included for variety.
4. Take *ume-sho-kuzu* twice a week.

Cerebral Allergies

Possible symptoms: Depression, neurosis, psychosis, schizophrenia, anxiety, dizziness, blurred vision, catatonia, paranoid delusions and hallucinations.

Possible triggers: Certain foods or chemicals.

1. Have some sea vegetables everyday.
2. Take *kombu* juice and *ume-sho-kuzu* twice a week each for one month.
3. As much as possible, use the vegetables whole, including the skins and tops.

Since allergies are caused by the buildup of excess, it is especially important not to overeat; take special care to chew very well, stop eating at each and every meal when you begin to feel full, and to wait about three hours after eating before you lie down to sleep.

At the same time, in order to let the extreme eruptions of allergies calm down, it is important to maintain a smooth elimination: if you become constipated, for example, or your menstruation isn't coming regularly, this can cause allergic symptoms to worsen. You can also be careful not to become generally too tight or tense (yang), as this can also prevent you from naturally discharging excess. Make sure to include lightly-cooked foods with a fresh taste everyday (especially with leafy vegetables), and to not overseason with salt (*miso, tamari* soy sauce, etc.) or overcook foods (beginners to macrobiotics often have this tendency).

If you become constipated, you can first give yourself a good, vigorous massage on the shoulders, legs and soles of your feet, as well as a light but firm massage in a circular motion (clockwise, in the direction of the colon) over the lower abdomen; also make sure to scrub your whole body everyday. And check to make sure you are chewing well. Then, if necessary, you can take the dish recommended above, agar-agar with barley malt or rice malt syrup. Sweet squash, boiled with grain sweetener and agar-agar, can also help relax tightened bowels. In cases of extreme constipation from hardened, impacted stools, you may take a tablespoon of heated raw sesame oil with several drops of fresh-grated ginger root juice added; or, an enema may be used.

For cases where your menstrual period is sluggish or has stopped, scrubbing your body is also helpful. Again, make sure your food is not overly salty, overcooked, or lacking in light, fresh-tasting dishes. Using a dried *daikon* leaf hip bath and special douche described later on is often helpful to relieve this problem. The lotus root, mustard and ginger compresses given above for respiratory problems have the same general purpose, to loosen and dissolve stagnated accumulations that can slow down your recovery.

Finally, how you hold yourself, move and express yourself also influence your ability to discharge freely and avoid accumulating excess energies. Make sure to keep yourself relaxed in mind and body, and to get some regular physical exercise to help keep all your energies moving. Regular mental exercise is also helpful, and you may engage in some form of regular expression, such as an art or other expressive activity.

4. Understanding Allergies ━━━━━

Being children of the universe, we are the natural heirs to everything around us. The universe never charges us rent for our stay on the earth, nor do we have to pay for the air, water, sunlight and the invisible world of thought and vibrations.

When healthy, we have a smooth exchange with our environment, taking in various nutrients and energies to continuously rebuild ourselves and giving back out what we can't use (in forms including bowel movements, urination, perspiration, exercise and activity).

When we eat, drink or otherwise take in some especially unusable or unhealthy part of our surroundings, such as very fatty foods or artificial drinks, our body automatically reacts to discharge it as quickly as it can. These strong discharging processes include such things as coughing, sneezing, running a fever, diarrhea, and others.

If we continue to accumulate excesses, the amount begins to exceed beyond our capacity to expel them immediately. We then store them in areas where they can get out easily including the lungs and bronchi, under the skin, in the sinuses, in the colon, and other locations. Then, especially when the excesses we consumed were more yin (such as milk, sugar or tropical fruit juices), we eventually may create a very strong contraction or tightening reaction (more yang) to counterbalance. These are the violent reactions of asthmatic attacks, allergic skin eruptions, vomiting, and other common symptoms of allergies. Allergies are our body's way of overreacting to normally mild irritants to compensate for our previous history of overconsumption. (A thorough explanation of how allergies develop is presented in the companion to this volume, *Allergies* by Michio Kushi.)

In particular, the foods that cause most allergies are: milk and all dairy products, overly oily and greasy foods, animal fat, sugar and other concentrated or artificial sweets and sweeteners, refined foods and flour products, tropical fruits, juices and vegetables with tropical origins (tomatoes, potatoes, eggplants, avocadoes, and others), and often various drugs, chemical additives, and other similar products. Among these, dairy foods, sugar and tropical fruits are probably the most common and prevalent causes.

In addition to avoiding the foods listed above, there are certain others that we would normally include in macrobiotics, but which are better to initially reduce or avoid temporarily when approaching allergies. These may include vegetable oils, temperate climate fruits, whole grain flour products, and so on depending on your particular allergy. After about two to three months you would gradually begin to broaden your diet to include the normal standard macrobiotic way of eating. Generally, most allergies will disappear or be substantially alleviated within three to six months of more balanced eating.

Eating macrobiotically is more than using "health foods"—actually, it is an expression of our respect for nature and of our harmony within it. Practically speaking, eating macrobiotically means that we no longer take in the kinds of excesses that create the accumulations that lead to allergies.

The hypersensitive, overreacting allergic stage disrupts our sense of being at peace with the world around us. Suddenly normally harmless things like cat fur, grasses or wheat become our enemies: we enter a state of seige. This feeling of war with nature actually underlies most of the actions, thoughts and "dog eat dog" attitudes of the modern world. The idea that we are foreigners at war with the rest of nature couldn't be further from the truth. Instead of merely attacking the *symptoms* of allergies, it is best to change the *cause* of the symptoms which is the imbalanced way that we eat, drink, think and live. If we accept everything around us, including our difficulties, as our friends, we not only help to alleviate allergies but also we gain more happiness, human freedom and a sense of belonging to the world.

5. Menu Planning ▬▬▬▬▬▬

When planning a menu, there are several things to consider.

1. The relative proportions of grain, vegetables, soup, beans, and so on in a meal as recommended in the standard dietary suggestions.
2. Adjustments for allergic conditions (see *Dietary Adjustment for Allergies* chapter).
3. Make sure that there is variety in your meals by varying:
   A. *The types of vegetables and grains used.* Everyday have some kind of root vegetable, fresh and leafy green and in some capacity, a small amount of sea vegetable. It is helpful to have brown rice everyday but there are many ways you can vary this basic dish as you will see in the menu examples.
   B. *The seasonings, condiments and pickles used.* (It is preferred that one has a small amount of pickles daily.)
   C. *The cooking methods employed.* Everyday, have some quickly boiled or blanched greens as well as pressure-cooked or longer time cooked items.
   D. *The sizes, shapes, colors and textures from dish to dish.* Use attractive garnishes to brighten your meals.
4. *Seasonal and climatic adjustments.* For hot weather, emphasize more fresh, lightly boiled or steamed vegetables, salads, less cooking time and less oil and salt. For colder weather, emphasize more hearty, rich dishes, stews and thick soups, protein such as found in beans, root vegetables and a little more salt and oil.
5. *Adjustments for the time of day.* Beans, hardy dishes, and stronger seasonings are best eaten for dinner. It is recommended that lunches and breakfasts be kept simple and light otherwise one may feel heavy and sluggish throughout the day. Soft porridges and whole grain cereals are delicious for breakfast.
6. *Adjustments for age.* For babies, younger children and elderly persons, serve more soft foods and sweet tasting vegetables with a minimum amount of seasonings. It is preferred that babies don't eat any salt at all. Teens and adults can have more seasonings and more crisp, solid vegetables.
7. *Lifestyle adjustments.* People doing more physical exercise, work and activities need more protein and hardy, rich dishes than someone who is more sedentary.

8. *Use as much of your leftovers as you can.* The menus below disregard leftovers to emphasize variety but normally a grain or bean dish, for example, can last for several days or more. Besides simply reheating your leftovers you can also rework them into a new format. For instance, last night's dinner rice can be this mornings soft rice. As another example, you can add a few pieces of *tofu* when reheating yesterday's root vegetables. The possibilities are endless. All this adds more appeal and variety to your meals.

One point that I particularly want to stress is that one should *Have Fresh, Quickly Boiled or Blanched Leafy Greens Everyday*. Therefore, boil only as much greens as you can have in one meal.

A General Seven Day Menu for Allergic Persons

	Breakfast	Lunch	Dinner
1	*Miso* Soft Rice *Bancha* Tea	*Udon* Noodles in Broth Boiled Cabbage Red Radish Quick Pickles *Mugicha* Tea	*Tamari* Broth Soup w/Onion & Fu Brown Rice, Pressure- Cooked *Azuki* Beans/Squash/ *Kombu* *Arame* w/Lotus Root, Leek & *Shiitake* Boiled Watercress Sauerkraut *Bancha* Tea
2	Barley Porridge w/*Gomashio* Grain Tea	Rice Balls Boiled Salad *Bancha* Tea	Lotus Seed Rice *Miso* Soup w/*Daikon* & *Wakame* Cabbage, Carrots & Seitan Boiled Collard Greens *Shio Kombu* *Mugicha* Tea
3	*Mochi* w/Grated *Daikon* *Miso* Soup w/Fresh *Tofu* & Watercress *Bancha* Tea	Millet/Squash Boiled Kale *Takuan* Pickles *Mugicha* Tea	*Tamari* Broth Soup w/Carrots & Onions *Azuki* Bean Rice Dried *Daikon* & *Kombu* Steamed Broccoli & Cauliflower Lotus Root Pickles *Bancha* Tea

4	Millet Porridge *Shiso* Leaf Condiment *Mugicha* Tea	*Arepas* Boiled Watercress Broccoli Stem *Miso* 　Pickles *Mu* Tea	Rice w/Rye Berries *Miso* Soup w/*Wakame* 　& Leeks *Arame*/Dried *Tofu*/ 　Carrots/Onions Boiled Chinese 　Cabbage Quick Pressed *Daikon* 　Pickles *Amazake* Pudding *Bancha* Tea
5	Plain Soft Rice 　w/*Nori* & *Umeboshi* *Miso* Soup w/Chinese 　Cabbage & Turnips *Mugicha* Tea	*Sushi* Boiled Mustard Greens 　& Carrots *Bancha* Tea	Millet/Squash Soup Sesame Seed Rice *Daikon*/Lotus/*Shiitake* 　*Nishime* Boiled Kale Cauliflower Pickles *Wakame* Powder Grain Coffee
6	Soft Rice w/*Miso* Chinese Cabbage Pickles *Bancha* Tea	Corn On The Cob w/ 　*Umeboshi* Boiled Broccoli *Mugicha* Tea	Lentil Soup Sweet Rice/Millet 　w/*Gomashio* *Kinpira* Carrots & 　Burdock *Wakame* & Ginger Boiled Chinese 　Cabbage/Watercress *Daikon* Top Pickles *Bancha* Tea
7	Creamy *Kasha* (Substitute Scotch Oats 　Porridge for Skin 　Allergies.) Sauerkraut *Mugicha* Tea	Boiled Couscous *Miso* Soup/Watercress/Fu Lotus Root Pickles *Bancha* Tea	Clear Fish Soup Rice with Barley Carrot/Lotus/Burdock 　*Nishime* Boiled Cauliflower & 　Broccoli Mustard Green Pickles Applesauce *Nori* Condiment Grain Coffee

Snacks: Rice Cakes, Roasted Peanuts, Leftovers, *Mochi*, Unbuttered Popcorn, Unsweetened Puffed Cereals, Roasted Pumpkin or Sesame Seeds with or without Raisins

6. Cookware ▬▬▬▬▬▬▬▬▬▬▬

Along with stocking the kitchen with good food, you need to equip it with a collection of essential cookware. Having the right tools in front of you makes all the difference in your cooking experience by freeing your mind to work with a more relaxed and creative attitude. This naturally has a profound effect on your well-being as well as affecting the quality, taste and appeal of your meals. Also, some types of kitchen equipment should best be avoided as they are suspected to be detrimental to your health, while others are a must for their beneficial influences. Listed below is a checklist of what you'll need.

1. We recommend a gas stove as opposed to an electric one. There are several reasons for this:

    A. Electricity dissipates the molecular structure and strength of your food by causing the electrons to bounce out of the atomic field and leaving the atom very unstable. Gas, on the other hand, just bounces the molecules around, while leaving them intact.

    B. It's very hard to fine tune your cooking with electricity. It is a conductive heat which first warms the coils and then the pot and its contents from the bottom up. You can't change the temperature quickly when turning to high or low because it takes some time to cool or heat the pot. It's difficult to cook uniformly and it's possible that the bottom can burn while the top needs more cooking. A gas flame heats the air around it instead. The food is cooked much more evenly and the temperature can be adjusted immediately (a pot of water will instantly stop boiling the moment you turn off the flame, for example). Meals are more well cooked.

    C. Because of these drawbacks in electric cooking, a person may not feel satisfied with the meal and may crave strong salt or animal food (to counter the yin and weakening effects) which in turn causes a craving for excessive sweets and other yin foods. In other words, it becomes more of a struggle to eat in a balanced manner and stay on the macrobiotic diet.

    A microwave oven is definitely out of the picture and should be avoided, particularly if you are sick. It zaps your food with radioactive waves at three billion cycles per second (a regular electric stove runs at 60 cycles per second and is actually a low form of radiation).

It disintegrates instead of cooks and can cause the same effect in your body. Not only does it not help you to regain your health but it is suspected by some people to contribute to illnesses. Recent studies have shown that it produces tumors in mice.

After gas, wood is the best source of heat (followed by coal or charcoal) though it is impractical for most modern homes. It has a peaceful energy and at the same time it gives great strength.

2. Several stainless steel pots of varying sizes. The steel doesn't interfere with the energies of the food. It's best to avoid aluminum because it is a poisonous substance and under high temperatures or when cooking very acidic (sweet) or alkaline (salty) foods, harmful toxins are released and mixed in with your ingredients.

Cookware made out of glass (like pyrex), earthenware, and enamelware are also excellent materials to cook in. (Be careful that you don't pour cold water into a heated enamel pot or leave it empty over a flame as this will cause it to crack. Let it cool off before you attempt to wash it. It is also easily scratched so don't clean it with a steel wool scrubber and use a wooden spoon when handling food inside it.)

3. At least one pressure-cooker (stainless or enamel steel). This is an ideal pot for cooking grains, beans, root vegetables (like big chunks of burdock), squash, or anything that takes a long-time to soften. The nutrients are better retained and everything is cooked more thoroughly, quickly and with more energy than when prepared in a regular pot.

To use, put ingredients inside (not more than ¾ full), cover (don't forget to put the weight attachment on top) and over a medium high flame, bring it up to pressure. You can tell it's up when there is a lot of hissing and the weight begins to jiggle and shake. Then, immediately turn down the flame and, if needed, place a heat deflector underneath. Simmer (anywhere from 5–10 minutes to an hour or more depending on what's inside) until the food is done. Take the pot off the stove and let the pressure come down. You can let it come down naturally or rinse the pot under cold running water in the sink. This brings it down right away.

I should add that before you cook, carefully take a good look at the cover. Inspect the hole (on which you place the weight) and make sure that it isn't clogged. Otherwise, an explosion can occur when the pressure is high. Also, look at the rubber rings on the inside of the lid and in the pot itself where the rings touch. Remove any bits of food or other substances which may be stuck there as they will create a gap where steam can escape and as a result, the pressure will never build up.

4. Several cast-iron skillets for roasting and sautéing. Season them when you first get them and from time to time thereafter. To do this, wash and dry them thoroughly. Rub sesame oil all over (outside also) with a paper towel. You can coat the inside by rotating and tilting the pan over a flame. Place them in the oven at 225°–250° F. for 2–3 hours. Then, let them sit for a few hours until they cool. Seasoning prevents the pans from rusting. For the same reason, don't soak them in hot, soapy water, and dry them thoroughly over a low flame after you wash them.

5. One deep cast-iron pot for deep-frying. Cast-iron is the best material to hold the intense heat of the oil.

6. Baking containers including pie plates, bread pans, muffin tins, and so on. Again, avoid aluminum.

7. An optional *wok* (a Chinese-style skillet). The cast-iron skillets can effectively cover your sautéing needs but a *wok* is great for quick, light and fast cooking vegetables and fish.

8. Several stainless steel mixing bowls in different sizes for washing and mixing your food.

9. Large wooden serving bowls for your grains. Wood gives your grains room to breathe as well as retarding their spoilage as they absorb any excess water. You need to oil the bowls periodically to prevent them from cracking. Heat some sesame oil, pour it into a completely dry bowl which you rotate until the inside is completely oiled. Oil the outside also, with a brush or paper towel. Let it sit for a few hours until it dries completely.

10. Various other attractive serving containers made of glass, china, or ceramics. (Plastic is to be avoided.)

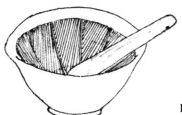

Fig. 5 *Suribachi* **and pestle**

11. A stainless steel or bamboo steamer.

12. A colander for rinsing noodles and other foods.

13. A fine strainer for washing seeds and grains.

14. A *suribachi* and pestle for making *gomashio* and other condiments. This is a Japanese ceramic bowl with grooves, made for crushing roasted sesame seeds, sea vegetables and so on.

15. A food mill for puréeing cooked grains and vegetables. (An electric blender is more disruptive to the energies of foods. Instead of using one on a regular basis I like to save it for parties or special occasions when working with large volumes.)

16. A grain mill for grinding grains and nuts into flour. Flour is best when used soon after grinding. It immediately starts to oxidize and begins to lose some of its nutrients. Also, it is most delicious when fresh. (Your local natural food store may have a good supply of flour as well.)

17. A pickle press for making pickles and pressed salads.

18. An earthenware crock with a wide mouth is good for making bran pickles among other things.

19. Tea pot or kettle. Avoid aluminum.

20. A tea strainer for straining out leaves and twigs when serving the tea. A bamboo one, found in natural food and Oriental stores is the best one to use.

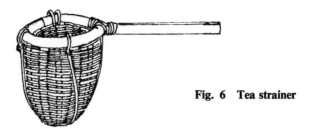

Fig. 6   Tea strainer

21. Large glass jars for storing grains, beans, nuts, seeds and other foods as well as for making pickles.

22. Wooden cutting boards. Keep a separate one for fish and animal foods as their bacteria can have a toxic effect on vegetables.

23. Knives. The square shaped Oriental knives are the easiest and the most efficient. They come in;
   A. carbon (which has a good sharp edge but rusts and chips easily),
   B. stainless steel (which doesn't rust but isn't as sharp), and
   C. high-grade carbon with stainless steel which doesn't rust and is sharp as well (but is more expensive).

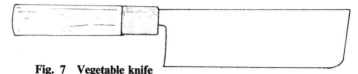

Fig. 7 Vegetable knife

To protect the carbon knives, wash them in warm, soapy water and dry them immediately, right after you use them. If rust starts to appear, scrape it off with a steel wool scrubber. Along with keeping your knives as dry as possible, they may be coated with a little sesame oil after use.

You will want to get a sharpening stone along with a knife to keep the edges of your knives sharp. Oil the stone with a vegetable oil or rinse it in water before you use it. Tilt the knife at a 20 degree angle and sweep the blade against the stone in several circular motions. You can use one of your hands to press down upon the blade while the other hand holds the knife and moves it in circles. Sharpen the entire length of the edge. You may choose to sharpen just one side for more control (the right side for right handers and the left side for lefties). Do not use this knife for bread as its blade may be destroyed.

24. A bread knife. The best knife for cutting bread has a long, thin blade with a serrated edge.

25. A grater, most often used for grating fresh ginger, *daikon*, carrots, onions, lotus root, *jinenjo*, and taro potato in macrobiotic cooking.

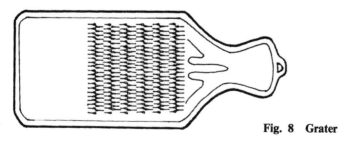

Fig. 8 Grater

26. A vegetable peeler, good for removing skins of cucumbers, apples and so on, when necessary.

27. A flame or heat deflector. This thin metal plate is placed under the pot or pressure-cooker to even the flame and to help prevent the food from burning. Don't use the white asbestos deflector as asbestos is poisonous.

28. An oil skimmer for lifting small bits of batter and food from *tempura* oil as well as for lifting vegetables from a pot of water.

29. A natural bristle brush for brushing oil into a skillet, cookie sheets, muffin tins, pie plates and so on. Any small, clean, unused brush can be used.

30. Drop tops. These tops fit inside the pot and sit directly on top of the food you are cooking, especially effective in cooking beans. They add some pressure but let steam escape and thus the food is cooked more thoroughly and softens more quickly.

31. Drop tops for pickles made in a keg such as bran pickles. A wooden one is the best. A heavy stone or weight is placed on top for pressure. A plate is a good substitute if a wooden one can't be found.

32. A vegetable brush with natural bristles is best for washing vegetables. They can be found in natural or Oriental food stores.

33. Wooden spoons for stirring, mixing, scooping and serving food before and after you cook. Wood has the best energy in interaction with your food as well as being more gentle to your pots, pans and bowls. Wooden spoons don't scratch cookware.

34. A bamboo rice paddle for handling and serving your grains.

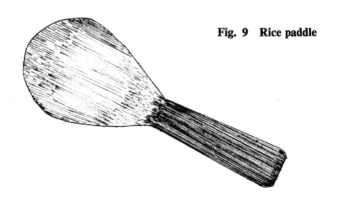

Fig. 9 Rice paddle

35. Soup ladles.

36. Rubber spatula for scraping batter, puréed food and so on from bowls and pots.

37. A metal spatula for turning food over.

38. Cooking chopsticks. These are longer than the table version.

39. A rolling pin.

40. Measuring cups and spoons.

41. Sushi mats for making *sushi* and covering cooked food. (They let air circulate and help retard spoilage).

42. Bamboo mats. Also for covering food.

43. 100 percent cotton cheesecloths, used as covers when making pickles and also for making little sacks to contain foods in cooking (sort of like a tea bag).

44. Paper towels.

7. Cooking Attitude

Besides the food and cookware, to be a good cook you need to have the right attitude and frame of mind. Here is another check list.

1. Leave all your worries, problems, and angers behind as you relax your mind and body into a peaceful, calm state of being. All your thoughts and emotions get mixed into the food and have an effect on anyone who eats it. Here are some things, among others, which you can think about as you cook:

    A. Pour your love and healing vibrations into your food and imagine that whoever eats it will become healthier and happier.

    B. Imagine that the food has the power to help realize everyone's dreams and that with this tool you have the ability to vitalize and inspire whole civilizations, because you do.

    C. In your mind, thank the farmer, trucker, store keeper, mother nature, the food itself, cookware companies and anyone else who has made it possible for you to have these wonderful ingredients and utensils in front of you.

    D. Imagine that you are composing a symphony or painting a masterpiece as you combine colors, textures, tastes and smells into beautiful and dynamic combinations. Release your creativity and intuition more and more, day by day.

    E. Realize that there is always more to learn. Don't ever become arrogant and think that you know it all. Be open and you can learn from everyone around you. We all have different perspectives and ideas and therefore we all have something to offer.

2. Clean and organize your kitchen and surroundings before, during and after you cook.

3. If you have long hair, tie it back to help prevent it from catching on fire as well as from falling into the food. Wear a clean apron and roll up your sleeves.

4. Work quickly, calmly and efficiently, economically making the most of your time. Avoid munching while you cook as this will really slow you down.

5. Keep other activities and distractions to a minimum and concentrate all your energies in your cooking.

6. When making your menu, first look at all your leftovers and older vegetables and use these first. Don't waste any food. Don't buy more perishables than you need. Look first at your supply before you go shopping.

7. Develop your intuition and common sense so that you can appropriately adapt your meals to the weather, the season, the people for whom you are cooking with their daily needs and changes, your own moods and any other influencing factors for that particular place and time.

8. Keep your meals simple. Don't mash together dozens of different ingredients into one dish. Go light on your seasonings and use them mainly to draw out and enhance the natural flavors of your food.

9. Decorate your food beautifully, set the table using appealing tableware, and make your dining area comfortable and aesthetically pleasing. This enhances your appetite and dining experience.

10. Take the time and place to relax, sit down and peacefully enjoy your meal with appreciation. Chew your food thoroughly, the saliva helps digestion. Also, it is best not to eat unless one is truly hungry.

8. Grains and Grain Products ━━━━━━━

The most helpful dishes for regular use include:

For Both Disorders:

> **Short-grain brown rice pressure-cooked**
> ***Azuki* rice**
> **Rice with lotus seeds**
> **Millet, rice with millet**
> **Soft rice with *nori* and *umeboshi***
> **Rice with whole rye berries**

Grains stored in a cool, dark, dry location can be kept forever. (Get them organic as much as possible.) To retain the maximum energy of your grains, leave grains unhusked until you cook with them if possible.

Before you wash grains, spread a handful at a time onto a plate and remove any stones and other debris which may be mixed in. Then, place the grains in a bowl (the lightweight stainless steel mixing bowls are excellent for this), cover with cold water and very gently stir and rinse off any dirt that floats to the top until the water becomes clear. Then, place the grain in a colander or strainer. (Wash quickly to help retain as many nutrients in the grain as possible.)

There are several kinds of grains that are available:

Brown Rice: ━━━━━━━━━━━━━━━━━━━━━━━━━━

Brown rice, being the easiest to digest, is the most suitable grain for daily use. You can have it everyday, regardless of whether you are in the transitional, healing or standard phase. We eat it at almost every meal. The other grains serve as variations, either as a substitute or as an additional ingredient in a meal. We mainly use four types of rice:

1. *Short-grain:* It is the variety with the hardiest taste and energy and the most effective one for creating a healthy balanced condition in your body. Use this one most of the time, especially in the winter.
2. *Medium-grain:* This is more soft and moist and is a nice variation.
3. *Long-grain:* This is light and fluffy, excellent for fried rice, and makes a great alternative in the summer and warmer climates.
4. *Sweet rice:* This is even more sweet and glutinous than the short grain and is quite sticky. This grain can be added to other grains periodically for a sweeter taste, and also serves as a base for *ohagi*,

mochi and *amazake.*

We recommend pressure-cooking your rice most of the time. This form of preparation cooks the grains more thoroughly, they become easier to digest, are less soggy, more sweet and more healing. Along with the help of a pressure-cooker there are two ways to make your grain softer, sweeter and more digestible;

1. *Non-soaking:* Start cooking the grain very slowly over a low flame, in an uncovered pressure-cooker. Don't put any salt in yet so that it will take more time to come to a boil. When it comes to a boil, add the salt, cover and bring it up to pressure (it is up when the gauge hisses). Then, place a heat deflector underneath (make sure the flame is on medium low) and simmer for 45–50 minutes.

2. *Soaking:* Soak the rice (covered with cold water) for 3–5 hours or overnight. Place in the pressure-cooker (along with the soaking water). This time, add salt and cover right away (otherwise it may turn out too soggy). Put on a medium high flame and bring it up to pressure. When it is up, turn the flame down to medium low, place a heat deflector underneath and simmer for 45–50 minutes.

Basic Brown Rice (Pressure-Cooked)
(Use everyday, the principle food for all conditions.)

3 cups organic brown rice
3 ¾–4 ½ cups spring water
3 pinches sea salt

Pressure-cook following one of the above methods. Let the pressure come down completely before removing the cover. Scoop out the rice with a wet rice paddle or wooden spoon into a wooden bowl as you separate and air out the lumps.

The bottom rice can be mixed in if it's not burnt. Keep the brown side turned down and totally covered to help keep it soft. If the bottom is really stuck to the pot, keep a 1″ layer of rice in the pot, put the lid back on, and let it sit for 20–30 minutes. The warmth of the fresh rice will help to loosen and soften the bottom.

Keep the rice covered with a bamboo or *sushi* mat. They protect it while letting it have air to breathe. Then dish the rice into individual bowls and serve. Serves 6.

There are many variations that you can use. Below are four helpful recipes followed by a partial listing of other variations.

Azuki Bean Rice
(Helps strengthen the kidneys and adrenals.)

  2½ cups brown rice
  ½ cup *azuki* beans
  4½ cups spring water
  3 pinches sea salt
  1 piece *kombu*, 3″–6″ long

Wash *azuki* beans and boil them with the *kombu* in 2 cups of water
for 10–15 minutes until the water becomes red. Cool the beans till
they are lukewarm. Wash the rice, put it in the pressure-cooker with
the beans and the red, boiled juice. Use pressure-cooking method
#1 (*Non-soaking*) and follow the directions for *Basic Brown Rice*. Or
you can soak the rice and beans together overnight and use method
#2 (*Soaking*). Serves 6.

Lotus Seed Rice
(The addition of lotus seeds makes this dish especially strengthening
for the lungs and the kidneys.)

  2½ cups brown rice
  ½ cup lotus seeds
  4½ cups spring water
  3 pinches sea salt

Wash and soak lotus seeds and rice 3–4 hours or overnight. Pressure-
cook using method #2 and following the directions for *Basic Brown
Rice* (*Pressure-cooked*). Serves 6.

Sesame Seed Rice
(Helps improve general vitality.)

  2½ cups brown rice
  ½ cup roasted white or black sesame seeds
  3¾–4½ cups spring water
  3 pinches sea salt

Wash and quickly roast white or black sesame seeds (being careful
not to burn them) in a skillet stirring with a wooden spoon until
a nutty fragrance is emitted. Combine with all the other ingredients
and cook as in *Basic Brown Rice* (*Pressure-cooked*). Serves 6.

Sweet Rice and Millet
(Strengthens spleen, pancreas and stomach.)

  2 cups sweet rice
  1 cup millet
  4 cups spring water
  3 pinches sea salt

Wash and combine all the ingredients and cook as in *Basic Brown Rice* (*Pressure-cooked*), method #2 (minus the *soaking*) for 40–45 minutes. Serves 6.

Other variations include:

1) 2½ cups rice + ½ cup barley (4½ cups water)
2) 2 cups rice + 1 cup millet (4½ cups water)
3) 2 cups rice + 1 cup sweet rice
4) 2½ cups rice + ½ cup wheat berries (soaked overnight)
5) 2½ cups rice + ½ cup chickpeas (soaked overnight)
6) 2 cups rice + 1 cup dried chestnuts
7) 2 cups rice + 1 cup fresh corn kernels (3 cups water)
8) 2½ cups rice + ½ cup wild rice
9) 2 cups rice + 1 cup *umeboshi* plum (instead of salt)
10) *Bancha* tea instead of water
11) 2½ cups rice + 1 cup squash
12) 2½ cups rice + ½ cup roasted black or yellow soybeans

You can also boil the rice once in a while, particularly for hypoglycemia. It doesn't give you the strength of pressure-cooking but it is a great alternative when you want something lighter, more yin and to add some variety. When you boil your rice, make sure to chew well. You can dry-roast the rice before boiling it for variation.

Basic Brown Rice (Boiled)

2 cups organic brown rice, washed
4 cups spring water
2 pinches sea salt

Put washed rice into a pot (preferably with a heavy lid) with water and salt. Bring to a boil, then lower the flame, place a heat deflector underneath and simmer for about 1 hour or until all the water has been absorbed. Wet a wooden spoon or rice paddle (so the rice won't stick to it) and dish out the rice into a wooden bowl. Keep covered with a *sushi* or bamboo mat. (*Option:* You can roast the rice in a skillet till golden brown before boiling it. This gives more flavor. Gently stir the grains in the skillet with a wooden spoon to prevent them from burning.) Serves 4.

When someone isn't feeling well, we often make soft rice. It is more soothing and is easier on the digestve system. A bowl of it is usually accompanied by an *umeboshi* plum which also helps digestion. Even if you are feeling well, this makes a delicious porridge. If you leave out the salt, this also makes a perfect food for babies and young children.

Soft Rice (Plain)
(A good healing dish.)

  1 cup brown rice
  5 cups water
  1 pinch sea salt

Cook as in *Basic Brown Rice* (*Pressure-cooked*). You can also boil it by simmering it overnight over a low flame and a heat deflector. If you do so, use 10 cups of water to every cup of rice. Serves 5.

People suffering from weak digestion could use a bowl of *miso* soup or a bowl of soft *miso* rice regularly. Below is a soft rice recipe made from cooked brown rice.

Ojiya (Soft Rice with *Miso*)
(Have often while healing.)

  2 cups leftover cooked brown rice
  4–5 cups spring water
  3 Tbsps. (or to taste) *miso* instead of salt
  1 strip *kombu* (about 4″–6″ long)
  3–4 sliced scallions

Wash, soak and slice the *kombu* and place it into the bottom of a pot or pressure-cooker. Add the rice and water and bring them up to a boil or to pressure. Turn the flame to low, place a deflector underneath and simmer or pressure-cook for ½ hour. Add 1 table-spoon or so of water to the *miso* and stir it in until the *miso* becomes a purée. Uncover the rice (wait until the pressure is gone if using a pressure-cooker) and then put it back onto the stove. Mix the *miso*, simmer for another 3–5 minutes and turn off the flame. Garnish with sliced scallions and serve immediately. Serves 4–5.

Rice Cream with *Nori* and *Umeboshi*
(Rice cream is a dish with special healing qualities. It helps purify blood and lymph.)

  1 cup dry-roasted brown rice
  3–6 cups spring water
  1 pinch sea salt
  1 toasted sheet of *nori*
  1 *umeboshi* plum
  Cheesecloth

Pressure-cook with sea salt and water for 1 hour following directions for *Basic Brown Rice* (*Pressure-cooked*). Make a sack out of clean cheesecloth. Cool off the cooked rice, place some inside the sack and squeeze out as much of the liquid cream as you can. Reheat and eat this with *nori* and an *umeboshi* plum. The leftover pulp can be eaten separately or added to soup or vegetable dishes. (Occasionally, instead of soaking the rice in the beginning you can dry-roast it in a skillet until golden brown.) Serves 2.

Musubi (Rice Ball)
(Great for lunches, picnics and trips, it is also a very strengthening, stabilizing way to eat rice.)

> 1 cup cooked short-grain (sticks well) brown rice
> 2 quarters of a *nori* sheet (a sheet cut in half and then half again)
> 1 pinch sea salt
> 1 *umeboshi* plum (or ½ if it's large)

Toast *nori* by passing it over an open flame a few times till it becomes green but not so much that it becomes crisp and crinkly. Tear it into 4 pieces.

Wet hands (to prevent the rice from sticking to them) in a bowl of salted water, put the rice in your palms and stick an *umeboshi* plum in the middle (the pit may be removed if desired). Tightly mold the rice around the plum into an English muffin shape or a flat triangle and put it down onto a plate.

Wash and dry hands. Then use a quarter of a sheet of *nori* on each side of the rice ball and cover with the shiny side (of the *nori*) on the outside. Firmly mold it on. You can then eat the rice ball or pack it up and take it on a trip to consume later. Serves 1.

Mochi is a traditional Japanese dish which is eaten on festive occasions. *Mochi* cakes or squares are made out of pounded sweet rice. Several pieces in *miso* soup can help strengthen the intestines.

Mochi (Homemade)

> 4 cups sweet rice
> 4 cups water
> 4 pinches sea salt
> A handful of any finely ground flour (pastry, sweet rice, arrowroot, etc.)

Cook as in *Basic Brown Rice* (*Pressure-cooked*). When done, in a wooden bowl, vigorously pound the rice with a large wooden pestle (which you wet initially and from time to time to prevent the rice from sticking to it) until all the grains are crushed and form a smooth, sticky mass. This may take a half hour. Sprinkle some flour onto a baking sheet and layer the rice on top (up to 1″ thick). Dry this for 1–2 days and then store it in the refrigerator.

When you want to have some, cut the *mochi* into small pieces and toast them in a skillet with or without oil until they become soft. This only takes a few minutes. (Turn them over when they are half done so that both sides toast evenly.) Serve them with some raw grated *daikon* with a few drops of *tamari* soy sauce added. The *daikon* helps in digestion of the *mochi*. Serves 5–6.

Fortunately, you can get previously pounded brown rice *mochi* in some natural food stores. All you have to do is to toast them for a few minutes.

Millet:

Millet is a more yang grain, being small, round, and more alkaline. It is good for the spleen and pancreas, it helps to settle an acidic stomach and it gives you warmth. For helping to relieve blood glucose disorders, it can be considered as a major grain after rice.

It cooks fairly quickly and comes out very soft so you can, but don't need to pressure-cook it. It can be made either light and fluffy or moist and creamy like a porridge. The fluffy style can be a little too dry, so it can often be eaten with a sauce or cooked with other ingredients. A standard combination uses squash (delicious). Other common companions are vegetables like carrots and onions as well as roasted seeds.

Millet (Dry)

   1 cup millet
   2 cups water
   1 pinch sea salt

Wash the millet. As an option, you may roast it with or without 1 tablespoon of oil in a skillet until a delicious nutty aroma is emitted. (Since allergic persons have to watch their oil content, dry-roast until your condition improves a bit. Stir quickly with a wooden spoon to prevent burning.) Bring the salt and water to a boil and slowly and carefully add the millet. Let this come up to a boil again. Then, cover the pot, turn the flame to medium low, place a heat deflector underneath and simmer for about 30 minutes. Serves 2.

Millet Porridge

   1 cup millet
   4 cups boiling water
   2 pinches sea salt

Bring salt and water to a boil. Wash the millet and carefully pour it into the pot of boiling water. Bring to a boil again, turn the flame to low, place a heat deflector underneath, cover and simmer for 30 minutes. Serves 3.

Millet and Squash

1 cup millet
½ cup buttercup or Hokkaido squash
2½ cups water
3 pinches sea salt

Wash and cut the squash into cubes. Remove the seeds and trim away the brown crusted substances on the surface of the skin, if there are any. If the skin happens to be extremely hard, you can slice it off (more a possible problem with the Hokkaido). Place the squash in a pot, put the millet on top, add water and salt, cover and bring to a boil. Then turn the flame to low, place a heat deflector underneath and simmer for 30 minutes. Serves 2–3.

Other variations:

1) Millet+cauliflower (3 ½ cups water)
2) Millet+squash+onions pressure-cooked 15 minutes.

Barley:

Barley is usually used in combination with other grains (such as rice) and vegetables. It is very mild tasting and lends itself easily to this. Cook it just like rice. It is light and has a cooling, calming energy, particularly helpful for hypoglycemia.

Barley Porridge

1 cup barley
4–5 cups spring water
1 pinch sea salt
Several parsley sprigs

Boil as in *Basic Brown Rice* (*Boiled*). Simmer for 1¼–1½ hours or until soft. Garnish with the parsley. Serves 5.

Buckwheat can grow in a very cold climate and has a short growing season. This grain gives strength, generates heat, and is good for the lungs, kidneys and bladder. It's a great winter food. However, people with hypoglycemia should use this grain only occasionally until their condition clears up.

Buckwheat can be cooked just like millet as it also cooks quickly and is a very soft grain. Below is a recipe for creamy *kasha* (buckwheat).

Creamy *Kasha*

>1 cup buckwheat groats
>2 scallions
>5 cups spring water
>1 pinch sea salt

Wash the buckwheat and put it into a pot. Add cold water and sea salt and bring to a boil. Then turn the flame down to low, place a flame deflector underneath and cook for 20–30 minutes. Wash and slice the scallions for a garnish. Serves 3.

Rye:

Rye, a hearty grain, is helpful for relieving allergies as it has often been found to be one of the easiest grains for allergic people to tolerate.

Rye with Rice

>2½ cups rice
>½ cup whole rye berries
>5 cups spring water
>3 pinches sea salt

Wash and soak the rye berries and rice for 3–5 hours or overnight.
Cook as in *Basic Brown Rice*. Pressure-cooked, for 50 minutes. Serves 6.

Rye with *Azuki* Beans

>2 cups rye berries
>½–¾ cup *azuki* beans
>5 cups spring water
>2 pinches sea salt

Wash and soak berries and beans together for 3–5 hours or overnight. Cook as in *Basic Brown Rice*, Pressure-cooked, for 60–70 minutes. Serves 6–8.

Oats:

Oats have more protein and fat than other grains. Therefore, while they are helpful to produce more warmth in the body, they shouldn't be taken on a daily basis as they can cause a buildup of mucus. Use about two times a week maximum during the initial healing stage.

You can buy whole oats, cut in half (called Scotch oats) or rolled (what we use for oatmeal). Rolled oats are the most mucus forming, so it is best to use them more occasionally.

Whole Oats

1 cup whole oats
5 cups spring water
1 pinch sea salt
1 strip *kombu* 3″–6″

Wash and soak oats for 3 hours. Add *kombu* (it helps to cut the fat in the oats) and pressure-cook 2 hours, or boil just like brown rice. If boiling, slowly simmer over a low flame for 3 or more hours or overnight. Serves 3.

Scotch Oats

1 cup Scotch oats
3 cups spring water
1 pinch sea salt
1 strip *kombu* 3″–6″

Combine water, salt and *kombu* and bring to a boil. Wash and dry-roast the oats in a skillet for 5 minutes, stirring with a wooden spoon over a medium low flame. Then, carefully pour them into the boiling water, bring up to a boil again, turn flame to medium low, place a heat deflector underneath, and cook for about 30–45 minutes. Serves 2.

Oatmeal (Rolled Oats)

Cook as in *Scotch Oats* but for a shorter time. Roast only 2–3 minutes (otherwise they will burn) and simmer for 20–30 minutes.

Wheat:

Wheat berries are harder to digest than other grains. They should always be soaked beforehand. Make sure you chew really well in order to insure good digestion.

Pressure-cook like rice except that you need to soak the berries for several hours or overnight. You also may need to cook them an extra 10–15 minutes. Use twice as much water as grain.

You can also get wheat in the form of bulghur, which has been partially boiled, dried and ground, or couscous, which has been refined and cracked. These forms enable you to cook wheat very quickly, especially couscous. These should not be staple foods as a lot of nutrients have been removed in the process. Use them as an occasional treat and variation.

Azuki Bean Wheat Berries

2 cups wheat berries
½–¾ cup *azuki* beans

4–5 cups spring water
2 pinches sea salt

Wash and soak berries and beans together for 3–5 hours or overnight. Pressure-cook as in *Basic Brown Rice*. Simmer for 60–70 minutes. Serves 6–8.

Bulghur and Vegetables

1 cup bulghur
¼ cup each of diced onions, carrots and celery
2–2½ cups spring water
1 pinch sea salt

Bring salt and water to a boil. Meanwhile, wash and dice the vegetables and layer them (onions on the bottom, then celery and finally carrots on top) into another pot. Add some water (just enough to cover the vegetables) and simmer until they are soft. Then, add the bulghur, pour the boiling water on top, cover and bring to a boil again. Turn the flame to low and simmer for 20 minutes. Serves 3.

Boiled Couscous

1 cup couscous
2½ cups spring water
1 pinch sea salt
Optional: 1 tsp. sesame oil

Bring the water, salt and optional oil to a boil. Pour in the couscous, turn the flame to low, cover and simmer for 5 minutes. Add some garnish or sauce. Serves 2.

Corn:

The corn eaten by the native American Indians was much harder, smaller and nutritious than most of the commercial corn available today. This grain was more effective in maintaining one's health, particularly strengthening the heart and blood vessels.

During the healing stage use only corn dishes that have been cooked whole at the beginning such as whole corn dishes and traditional *masa*, *tortillas* and so on. Avoid dishes that have been ground previous to any cooking as they may cause a buildup of excess mucus.

There are five main types of corn available today:

1. *Sweet corn*—The regular corn on the cob.
2. *Dent corn*—Corn with dented kernels used for making cornmeal.
3. *Flour corn*—Starchy variety used in Latin American cooking.
4. *Flint corn*—Starchy variety used in Latin American cooking.
5. *Popcorn.*

Corn on the Cob (Boiled)

Desired number of ears of fresh corn
A pot of water
Several pinches sea salt
1 Tbsp. *umeboshi* **paste**

Trim away the dry, outer leaves of the corn but keep the fresher inner wrapping intact. Chop off the excess straggly husk ends and silk hairs on the top end of the corn. Put sea salt in the water and bring the big pot up to a boil. Drop the corn in and boil for about 10 minutes. Take out the corn and serve. After unhusking your individual ear of corn, you can rub *umeboshi* paste on it (as you would with butter) if you want. Strain out any leftover silk hairs in the liquid with an oil skimmer and use this liquid for soup stock.

Dried Whole Corn (Dent, Flint or Flour)

2 cups whole, dried corn
8 cups spring water
2 pinches sea salt
1 cup sifted wood ash

Wash and soak the corn overnight. Put the corn, 4 cups of water and the wood ash (no salt) in a pressure-cooker. Cook for 30–45 minutes. When the corn is done, put it into a colander or strainer. Rinse out all the ash and remove the corn skins. (If the skins aren't loose enough, cook again with more ashes for another 10 minutes.) Pressure-cook the unhulled corn for 1 hour in a clean pot with salt and 4 more cups of water. You can serve this as it is or use this as a base for other corn recipes. Serves 4–6.

Masa (Corn Dough)

4 cups whole dried, flint or flour corn
8–10 cups water initially and 8 more cups later
1 cup sifted wood ash
3–4 pinches sea salt

Follow the directions in *Dried Whole Corn* except that you use 8–10 cups of water in the beginning and 8 more cups after the corn is hulled. Take out and cool the corn. Grind it in a hand grinder (not a blender). Knead this for about 15 minutes. You can moisten it with a little water if it is too dry. If you don't use the dough immediately, store it in the refrigerator (up to a week). This is the base for many corn recipes such as *arepas*, *tortillas*, cereals, and so on.

Arepas

> 3 cups *masa* corn dough (see above recipe)
> Boiling water
> Water to help shape the dough
> 2–3 pinches sea salt
> 1 Tbsp. sesame oil
> *Optional:* $\frac{1}{2}$ cup roasted sesame seeds

Knead the dough while mixing in salt and optional sesame seeds. It should feel like bread dough. If it's too dry, add a little water and if too wet, add more dough or let it sit and dry for a few minutes. Separate it into balls which you mold into English muffin shapes, except a little flatter. Boil some water, put the balls inside and remove them when they rise to the top. Heat some oil in a skillet, place the *arepas* inside, cover and cook them over a low flame for about 15–20 minutes. (Turn them over halfway through to cook the other side.) If you want, you can then slit them open and stuff them with beans and/or vegetables. Serves 4–6.

Grain Products:

During healing, it is generally recommended that you avoid flour products. This is especially so for baked items such as breads, pastries, pies, cookies, crackers and the like as they can cause mucus buildup. However, a few boiled products once in a while can be used without any detriments, as boiled foods are more digestible. This category includes whole wheat or buckwheat noodles, *fu* and *seitan*.

1. Noodles are a great snack and cook up very quickly. There are several types which are now available in most natural food stores.

   A. *Soba*—Long, thin, Oriental buckwheat noodles.
      1) Buckwheat with/without wheat in varying amounts
      2) *Jinenjo soba* (contains *jinenjo* flour)
      3) *Ito soba*—Extra thin and light
      4) *Ramen*—Instant noodles

   B. *Udon*—Long, Oriental wholewheat noodles
      1) Thicker than *soba* and contains wholewheat and sometimes unbleached, sifted white flour.
      2) *Somen*—Very thin wheat noodles
      3) *Ramen*—Instant noodles

   C. *Pasta*—Wheat alone or in combination with other grain flours.
      1) Spaghetti
      2) Shells

3) Spirals
4) Elbows
5) Ribbons
6) Ziti
7) Rigatoni
8) Linguini
9) Lasagna
10) Alphabets, etc.

Buy these noodles, especially the *ramen* and *pasta*, from natural food stores. The *ramen* bought in Oriental shops may contain animal fats, sugar, MSG, chemicals, additives and food coloring. *Pasta* bought in a regular store usually contains eggs which are best avoided.

To cook noodles, place them in a large pot of boiling water. (Too little water causes them to clump together.) As you put them in, stir and separate the noodles with a long chopstick to prevent them from lying side by side in a parallel fashion, otherwise they will stick together. (This precaution is basically for long thin noodles such as *udon* and *soba*.)

You can keep the flame high and add a little cold water each time the pot comes to a boil until the noodles are soft (usually about 3 times). Or you can turn the flame down a bit after adding the noodles and simmer until they are cooked. The first method is preferred as the noodles come out more firm and crisp. When done, the inside is the same color as the outside. Then, drain them in a colander and immediately run cold water over them. This helps to keep them from clumping together.

Don't make them too soggy especially if you are later going to reheat or fry them. Pay special attention to the *somen* and *ito soba* as they cook up very quickly and are absolutely horrible when soft and mushy.

Add a pinch of salt when boiling pasta. (*Udon* and *soba* already contain salt so they don't need it.) The leftover noodle water can be used in soup stocks.

After *ramen* is boiled, it is generally left in the pot and the accompanying packet of dry soup ingredients is mixed in. Read what the packet contains to make sure that the contents are healthy.

Noodles in Broth

1 pack *udon* or *soba* noodles previously boiled
1 3"–4" piece of *kombu*
2 *shiitake* mushrooms, soaked and sliced
4 cups water including *shiitake* soaking water
½ cube *tofu* cut into smaller cubes
3–5 Tbsp. *tamari* soy sauce

1–2 sheets toasted *nori*, cut into small pieces
3 chopped scallions

Make a soup stock by bringing *kombu, shiitake* and water to a boil and simmering for 5 minutes. Take out the *kombu* and *shiitake*. Boil the *tofu* and take them out when they rise to the top. Add the *tamari* soy sauce and simmer for 5–7 minutes. Put in some noodles (only add what you are immediately going to eat and keep the rest aside) until they become warm, then dish them out into individual bowls. Place some *tofu, shiitake* slices, *nori* and scallions on top of each one, pour some broth over them and serve.

For variation:
1) Use any combination of *shiitake, kombu* or bonito flake soup stocks.
2) Add different kinds of sea vegetables, root or green vegetables into the broth (they can be left in once they are put in), boil them till they are soft and add the *tamari* soy sauce.
3) Add different kinds of sea vegetables, root, green, boiled, sautéed, or raw (thinly sliced) vegetables as a garnish on top. Roasted seeds, *fu* (soak and boil it in the broth previously as was done with the *tofu* above), cooked *seitan* and *tempeh*, and grated *daikon* or ginger can also be added.
4) As a general rule, you can add anything as long as there is some kind of sea vegetables present as well as some kind of pungent item in the garnish. This would include scallions, diced raw onions, chives and grated ginger or *daikon*. (They help digestion.)

Zaru Soba

Soba, previously boiled
1 Tbsp. *tamari* soy sauce
1 Tbsp. brown rice vinegar
4 Tbsps. *kombu* soup stock
Chopped scallions
Nori, toasted and cut into thin strips

Place *soba* noodles onto an individual serving plate and place a few strips of *nori* on top. (In Japan they have special individual bamboo serving "plates" which allows the *soba* to drain.) Combine *tamari* soy sauce, rice vinegar, *kombu* stock, scallions into a small bowl to make a dip for the noodles. Make a dip for each person.

Macaroni with Carrots and Corn

> **2 cups of elbow, ziti, shell, spiral, ribbon or alphabet macaroni, previously boiled**
> **1 cup fresh corn off the cob** •
> **1 cup thinly quartered carrots**
> **3 pinches sea salt**
> **2 cups boiling water**
> **1 Tbsp. *kuzu* dissolved in a little water**
> ***Tamari* soy sauce to taste**
> **Several parsley sprigs**
> **¼ cup dry-roasted sesame seeds**

Put salt in the water and bring to a boil. Add and boil the corn kernels for several minutes until they are cooked. Scoop them out with an oil skimmer and add and boil the carrots until they soften. Take them out and combine with the corn and pasta in a serving dish.

Add *kuzu* to the pot of water and stir until it becomes transparent. Add *tamari* soy sauce to taste, stir and simmer another 2–3 minutes and pour the liquid over the pasta and vegetables. Sprinkle the sesame seeds on top, garnish with parsley sprigs and serve. Serves 4–6.

2. *Seitan* is made from the gluten of hard whole spring or winter wheat flours (they contain the most gluten). *Seitan* is protein rich.

Seitan

(This can also be bought in natural food stores. Avoid ones that have been heavily spiced if you are healing.)

> **3½ lbs. whole wheat flour (spring or winter)**
> **8–9 cups of water**

Place the flour into a large stainless steel mixing bowl, gradually add the water, form a dough and knead it for 5–15 minutes until it becomes stiff and earlobe consistency.

Submerge the dough in water and let it sit for 5–10 minutes. Then knead and separate the dough in the water until the liquid is full of bran and starch.

Drain the *seitan* in a colander which you place inside a large pot. (If you want, save the soaking water, starch and bran. It can be used to thicken soups, sauces, stews, puddings and so on as well as for pancakes, waffles, and sourdough starter.) Add cold water to the pot and start to knead all the bran out of the gluten.

If this water also becomes overly branny, add fresh water. (You may save this bran water as well, if you like.) Start to take small pieces of the gluten at a time and wash the bran out of them one by one. You can run them under the tap. (Some remaining flecks of bran here and there is OK. You don't have to worry about trying to get it perfectly branless.)

When finished, separate the gluten into several pieces and drop them into a pot of boiling water until they rise to the surface. (Or you can deep-fry them until they puff up and turn golden brown. Try it this way when no longer healing. It is delicous.)

You can cook the *seitan* further if you want. Put a piece of *kombu*, *seitan*, 1/3–1/4 cup *tamari* soy sauce and 6 cups of water into a pot, bring to a boil, turn flame to low, cover and simmer for about a half an hour. Eat as it is or add to other dishes including soups, salads, vegetables, stews, grains, and the like.

Seitan Stew

1 lotus root, cut into 1/4″ rounds
1 *daikon*, cut into 3/4″ rounds
5 *shiitake* mushrooms, soaked
Seitan, kombu, tamari mixture from the above recipe
Finely chopped parsley

Take the mixture from the above recipe, place the lotus root, *daikon* and *shiitake* mushrooms inside, add enough water so that it is level with or just covering the vegetables, bring to a boil, cover, turn flame to low and simmer 20–30 minutes or until the vegetables are soft. Add a cup or two of the leftover *seitan* starch water (see above recipe), and stir (to prevent burning) until the stew thickens. Garnish with the parsley and serve. Serves 5–7.

Cabbage, Parsnips and *Seitan*

2 cups cabbage, cut into 1″ squares
1 cup parsnips, sliced on a thin diagonal
Several pieces *seitan*
Enough water to cover the vegetables halfway
3 pinches sea salt
Tamari soy sauce to taste if needed

Place all the ingredients into a pot, bring to a boil, cover, turn flame to low and simmer for 10–15 minutes until the vegetables are soft. Serves 6.

3. *Fu* is also a by-product of wheat gluten. It looks like a cracker and is packaged and available in natural food stores. You can get *fu* in flat sheets or thick rounds which are available in small or large sizes.

Round *Fu*/*Daikon* and Greens/*Wakame*

1 *daikon*, cut into ½″ rounds
The greens of the *daikon* cut into ¼″ pieces
½ cup *wakame*, soaked and sliced into 1″ slices
1 package small round *fu*, soaked for 10 minutes
1 pinch sea salt
Pureed *miso* to taste

Layer *wakame*, *fu* and *daikon* into a pot, add salt and enough water to just cover the *fu*, cover, bring to a boil, turn flame to low and simmer. Before the *daikon* is completely softened, add the greens. When soft, uncover, boil away excess liquid, add the *miso*, and simmer another 5 minutes. Serves 4.

Flat *Fu* Soup with Carrots

1 cup carrots, cut into ¼″ rounds
½ cup carrot tops, finely minced
3–4 sheets flat *fu*, soaked & cut into ¼″ strips
2 pinches sea salt
3 tsps. pureed *miso* or 3 Tbsps. *tamari* soy sauce

Bring *kombu* stock to a boil and add the carrot tops until they soften and turn a bright green (a couple of minutes—depending on how small they are). Skim them out with an oil skimmer and put them aside for now.

Add salt, bring to a boil again, put in the carrots and *fu* strips and boil them until they soften. (The *fu* only takes about 3–5 minutes.) Add the *miso* or *tamari* soy sauce, simmer over a low flame for 2–4 minutes and serve, garnished with boiled carrot tops. Serves 6–8.

4. *Sourdough bread.* When healing, it is best to abstain from baked flour products as mentioned before, but if you do crave some, natural unyeasted sourdough bread is best.

Yeast is not recommended as it can cause indigestion and weakens the intestines.

Hard spring or winter wheat flours makes the best bread as they contain much gluten which helps the bread rise. Any other flour can be added in smaller proportions for a variation in taste as can any cooked grains. (Cooked grains that have already gone sour can replace the sourdough starter.)

Before making a sourdough bread, you at first need to make a starter.

Sourdough Starter

1 cup whole wheat flour
1–1 ½ cups well or spring water

Put flour and water into a bowl and mix them into a thick batter or porridge-like consistency, adding more flour or water if you need to. Cover with a damp towel and let it sit for 2–4 days at room temperature. When it bubbles and becomes sour, it is ready to use.

Sourdough Bread (2 Loaves)

5 cups whole wheat flour
1 cup sourdough starter (or sour *seitan* water)
2 cups water
1 tsp. sea salt

Mix the starter, water and 2½ cups (a half) of the flour, let sit uncovered in a warm place for an hour or so until it rises.

(At this point, you can save half of this batter for an ongoing starter which you can keep using, adding to and recycling every week; the longer it's been around the better the bread. If you don't want to bake one week, mix in a few spoonfuls of flour and water just to keep it going and to prevent it from spoiling. This should be stored in the refrigerator.)

Add the salt and remaining flour, form into a dough, and on a floured board, start kneading the bread, about 350–400 times. The more it is kneaded the better it will rise as the bread gets more and more elastic, glutinous and smooth. This is the secret to non-yeasted breads.

Place dough into a lightly oiled bowl, cover with a damp towel and let it sit overnight at room temperature.

The next morning, punch the dough down, knead it for a few minutes and divide it in half. Place the halves into a couple of oiled bread pans and with a knife make a lengthwise slit down the center of the tops. The slit helps to give the bread some room to grow and lets steam escape. Place them in a very warm place and let sit for another 2–3 hours or until the bread rises and the slits begin to open.

Make the slits deeper and take an oiled rubber spatula and pull the bread away from the sides of the pans. Bake at 350°–375° F. for about an hour until the bread forms a beautiful brown crust.

Insert a chopstick or fork into the bread and pull it out again. If no flour sticks to it, the bread is done. Also, when tapping the bottom, you will hear a hollow sound if the bread is finished. Remove from the pans and let the loaves cool on a bread rack for a couple of hours. Eating the bread while it's still hot may cause an upset stomach. Keep loaves in a cool, dark place, wrapped in a clean cotton cloth or towel.

Slice with a bread knife. If the bread becomes hard, you can steam the slices you want to eat for a few minutes. They then become moist and appear freshly baked.

9. Soups ━━━━━━━━━━━━━━━━━━━━━━

Most helpful soups for regular use include:

Miso soup with *kombu* or *wakame* and vegetables
Tamari broth soup with fibrous leafy vegetables (kale, watercress, *daikon* leaves, etc.)
Millet or rice soup with sweet-tasting or hard root vegetables (lotus root, burdock, etc.)
Azuki or lentil soup

Soup at the beginning of a meal prepares your digestive system for all the following dishes. Just about anything can be put into a soup. Practically all types of grains, beans and their products, vegetables, sea vegetables, and occasionally fish can be used.

Soups can be adapted seasonally (and be either warming or cooling) and can add contrast to the rest of the meal. There are some general guidelines on deciding what kind of soup to use.

In the winter, make more hearty stews and thick soups with more root vegetables, grains or beans and use more salt. In the summer make lighter soups with less ingredients and more liquid, more greens, *tofu*, and so on. Also make a greater use of clear or a light *tamari* broth soups in hot weather.

Care should be taken to balance the soup with the rest of the meal. Some examples are:

1. Make a bean soup for a light meal lacking in more protein-rich dishes such as beans, *tempeh*, or *natto*.
2. Make a sweet vegetable soup (squash, carrots, parsnips) if the meal is lacking this sweet taste.
3. Make a root vegetable soup if the meal is mostly greens and vice versa.
4. Make a grain soup to balance a more light meal.
5. Use finely chopped vegetables if the meal contains all big chunks and vice versa.
6. Use a color in the soup which is not represented in the meal.
7. If you are not making *miso* soup, you can add *miso* somewhere else in the meal.

Use a ladle to serve your soups. This can be kept on a plate on the counter next to the soup pot or in a bowl during the course of the meal, ready to be used whenever needed.

Especially during the first few months, it is recommended that everyday, one of your meals should contain *miso* soup (unless you have soft *miso* rice that day). Also everyday, at least one of your soups should contain sea vegetables. Garnishes are important (parsley or scallions) to balance your soups as well as for decoration.

1. *Miso soup:* *Miso* is an indispensable part of the macrobiotic diet. It gives vitality, strengthens the digestive system and blood quality, and improves your assimilation of carbohydrates. When healing, eat a small amount everyday, particularly in *miso* soup.

    Miso is very salty so care must be taken to avoid consuming too much of it at one time. To use, add a spoonful of water to a couple of tablespoons or more of *miso* and mix it in to make a purée. Then, add this to the soup (or any other dish calling for *miso*).

    Miso should be added at the end after all the ingredients have softened and generally shouldn't be boiled as otherwise many valuable healing enzymes are destroyed. However, it is important to note that the soup must be simmered for a few minutes after the *miso* is added to help assimilate it into the body. If this isn't done, tightness can arise.

    The recipes below are for *hatcho* or *mugi* (barley) *miso*.

Basic *Miso* Soup

Wakame or kombu, soaked and sliced
Choice of vegetables
Puréed miso
Water
Scallion or parsley garnish

Soak *wakame* or *kombu* for 10 minutes and slice. Boil the slices in water, cutting your vegetables in the meantime. Add the vegetables to the boiling water and cook until they are soft. Dilute and purée the *miso* with some of the soup water, turn down the flame, and when the soup has stopped bubbling, gently add and stir the *miso* purée into the soup. Simmer for 2–4 minutes and serve with a garnish. It is important that the soup be light and energetic by keeping your vegetables fresh and crispy, being careful not to overcook them.

Wakame and *Daikon Miso* Soup

½ cup *wakame,* washed, soaked & sliced
½ cup *daikon* cut any way you want
4 cups spring water
1½ Tbsps. puréed *miso*
2 scallions sliced

Follow the recipe for *Basic Miso Soup*. Serves 6.

Chinese Cabbage and Turnips *Miso* Soup

½ cup Chinese cabbage, sliced into 1″ slices
½ cup turnips, sliced into thin half-moons
1 strip *kombu*, 4″ long, soaked & cut into matchsticks
4 cups spring water
1½ Tbsps. pureed *miso*
Several sprigs parsley garnish

Boil the *kombu* until it becomes soft. Then add the vegetables and cook as in *Basic Miso Soup*.

2. *Clear broth or tamari soy sauce soup:* This is a light soup which is very appealing in the hot summer months or when the rest of the meal is more heavy. A stronger *tamari* broth is very good as a standard supper soup or for noodles.

For a clear soup, make a soup stock (a few examples are listed at the end of this chapter) and add the vegetables and some form of salt. You may . . .

A. keep the clear color of the soup stock by using sea salt (a pinch or two for every cup of liquid),
B. make it darker with 2–3 tablespoons of *tamari* soy sauce for every four cups of liquid (most often used),
C. or use 1 tablespoon of *umeboshi* paste or 2–3 tablespoons of *umeboshi* vinegar or 2–3 *umeboshi* plums for every 4 cups of liquid. This gives an attractive pink coloring to your soup.

Daikon/Daikon Greens *Tamari* Broth Soup

½ cup thin *daikon* round
½ cup *daikon* tops, cut into 1″ slices
1 strip *kombu*, 4″–6″ long
4 cups spring water
2–3 Tbsps. *tamari* soy sauce

Make a *kombu* stock by boiling the *kombu* for 5 minutes. Remove the sea vegetable and add the *daikon* greens to the boiling water until they turn a bright green. Scoop out the greens with an oil skimmer and put them aside to drain in a colander for the time being. Boil the *daikon* rounds until they become soft. Add the *tamari* and simmer for 3–5 minutes. Pour the soup into individual serving bowls, garnish with the *daikon* greens and serve. Serves 4.

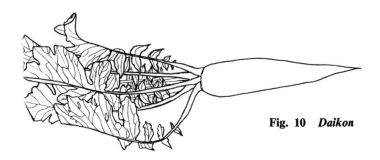

Fig. 10 *Daikon*

3. *Grain and bean soups:* You can pressure-cook these soups first or just boil them gently for a longer time.

A. To boil, layer the vegetables into a pot. Place the more yin vegetables on the bottom and more yang ones on the top (except for greens which are added later and placed on top of everything). Then add the grains or beans and enough water just to *Barely* cover everything. Bring to a slow boil, adding more water as the grains or beans expand. You can place a heat deflector underneath to help prevent burning. This is the same method used in boiling beans (see *Beans and Bean Products* chapter) except that instead of boiling away the excess liquid in the end, we add more to make it soupy. The salt and/or *miso* or *tamari* are added after the grain or bean has softened (simmer another 3–10 minutes after the seasoning is added). More water can be added if the consistency is too thick.

Soaking the bean or grain beforehand shortens the cooking time. You can also use previously cooked grains or beans. In this case, first boil the vegetables until they are soft before adding them. Also, you may sauté the vegetables and/or roast the grains or beans beforehand. An optional piece of *kombu* may be added in the bottom of the pot.

Millet/Burdock/Leek Soup

½ cup millet
¼ cup burdock, diced
½ cup leeks, cut into thin slices
5–6 cups spring water
½ tsp. sea salt
Several sprigs of parsley garnish

From the bottom up, layer the burdock, leeks and millet, and add sea salt and enough water to just cover them. As the millet expands, keep adding water little by little until it becomes soft. Then add more water if you want a soupier consistency. Serve with parsley. Serves 6.

Rice/Lotus Root Soup

> 1 cup cooked brown rice
> 1 lotus root, sliced into thin half-moons
> 1 piece *kombu*, 3″–6″ long
> 4 cups spring water
> 2 pinches sea salt

Put *kombu*, lotus root and sea salt into a small pot. Add a little water and boil the lotus root until it is soft. Add the rice and the rest of the water, bring to a boil, turn flame to low, place a heat deflector underneath, and simmer for 10–15 minutes. Serves 4.

B. Pressure-cooking. The grains or beans are first pressure-cooked. The cover is then taken off. The salt (especially in the case of beans as some grain dishes can take salt from the beginning), *tamari* soy sauce or *miso*, and perhaps some vegetables are then added. Then all this is simmered, up to 20–30 minutes longer, depending on the dish.

Azuki Bean/Lotus Seed Soup

> 1 cup *azuki* beans, soaked overnight
> ½ cup lotus seeds, soaked overnight
> ½ cup onions, diced
> 5–6 cups spring water
> ½ tsp. sea salt
> 1 strip *kombu*, 4″–6″
> Several sprigs of parsley garnish

Soak the lotus seeds and *azuki* beans together for several hours. Put them in a pressure cooker above the *kombu* and onions, add water and pressure-cook for 45 minutes after the pressure has come up. When done let the pressure come down, remove the cover, add the sea salt and simmer for another 10 minutes. Serve with parsley sprigs. Serves 6.

4. *Soup stocks:* These soup stocks can be used for any of the above types of soups. They are particularly good for the clear, *miso* and vegetable soups.

Kombu Soup Stock

1 piece *kombu*, 3"–6"
5–6 cups of water

If there is any dust on the *kombu*, wipe it off with a clean, damp cloth. Leave the white powder on. Bring the *kombu* and water to a boil, simmer about 3 minutes and remove the *kombu*. It can be reused for another stock (boil it longer the next time to get more out of it), added to another dish, or sliced and used in this one.

Other variations:

a) 4 *shiitake* mushrooms, simmer 5–6 minutes
b) 2 Tbsps. bonito fish flakes, 3–4 minutes
c) Any combination of *kombu, shiitake* and bonito
d) Odd and ends of vegetables such as onion skins, cabbage cores, roots, tops and so on. Wash well, boil 5 minutes, and discard or use for compost
e) Other sea vegetabes like *wakame* and dulse
f) Dry-roast grains such as rice, sweet rice, millet, buckwheat or barley until a nutty fragrance is emitted and use for stock. Simmer 4–5 minutes.
g) *Chirimen iriko* (small, whole dried fish available in natural and Oriental food stores).
Boil 2 Tbsps. for 3–4 minutes.
h) Leftover liquid from boiling vegetables
i) Water leftover from cooking beans
j) Diluted water leftover from cooking *seitan.*

10. Vegetables ▬▬▬▬▬▬▬▬▬▬▬

Most helpful dishes for regular use include:

Nishime style vegetables, especially with hardy roots like *daikon*, burdock, lotus, carrots, etc.)
Dried *daikon* with *kombu*
Hard leafy greens (kale, watercress, etc.), boiled or steamed
Boiled carrot, *daikon*, turnip or dandelion together with their greens
Any macrobiotic pickles which have been pickled longer than a week

For Asthma and Hay Fever:

A special emphasis on root vegetables

For Food Allergies:

Daikon or hard leafy greens pickled in *miso* and/or bran, pickled dried shredded *daikon*

As much as possible, you should get organically grown, chemical-free vegetables. Besides being healthier for you, they are more delicious. Organic farmers put much care and attention into producing food that benefits both mankind and the planet. Also avoid dull colored, limp, yellow leaved, soft spotted and wrinkled items as they are either too old, spoiled, dried up and/or don't have much vitality.

Choose locally grown produce as often as possible, though in the north during the winter you would have to rely more on southern grown ones. Prepackaged items tend to spoil more quickly. Stay away from canned and frozen foods. They have no energy and/or have added salt, sugar and preservatives, all of which are best avoided. Also, be careful not to buy waxed items.

At home, immediately remove any yellow leaves and spoiled parts of your vegetables before you store them. This helps to preserve the rest for a longer time. When storing vegetables in the refrigerator, keep them in a paper bag; this allows them to absorb extra moisture and thereby retards spoilage. A plastic bag retains water, doesn't allow your vegetables to breath and causes them to grow soggy and spoil more quickly. Keep your vegetables separated from your fruits for better preservation.

Don't wash your vegetables until you are ready to use them. Any soil left on them helps to keep them longer. When you do wash them, particularly your leafy greens, it helps to submerge them in a big bowl of water.

Swish them around a little bit and wash each leaf individually. This automatically separates and loosens the sand, soil and dirt which settles to the bottom of the bowl, as the greens stay afloat. This is much more effective and easier than just trying to rinse them under the tap. Roots can be scrubbed gently with a vegetable brush (*tawashi*) to remove the soil but make sure to keep the skin on. (If you are dealing with organic vegetables, you don't have to peel your cucumbers, carrots and so on as they are not sprayed, or covered with wax. The skins contain many nourishing nutrients.)

To wash leeks, cut them in half lengthwise and clean out all the dirt trapped in between the layers of leaves. The soil usually collects in the section where the colors change from white to green.

Always use cold water when you clean as hot water washes out many vitamins and minerals. Wash vegetables quickly. Soaking for any length of time also depletes valuable nutrients.

Within one dish, cut your vegetables uniformly for even cooking. Within a meal have a variety of different sizes represented in several dishes—smaller for sautéed items and bigger chunks for stews, for example.

Save the tops and roots of vegetables as much as you can. They can be cleaned, chopped very finely and incorporated into your vegetable dishes. You can also leave them uncut and use them in a soup stock. Using the whole plant helps to create a balance in your system.

I recommend the square, Japanese vegetable knives (see *cookware* section) for cutting your vegetables. They are very handy, flexible and easy to use. With these knives, don't cut straight down or use them like a saw. Starting with the front tip or edge, gently slide the length of the blade across your vegetables in one smooth stroke. *Important: Always Keep Your Fingertips Curled Underneath So That Your Knuckles Show When You're Cutting.* This helps to protect them from accidental cuts and slips and you also get a better grip on the vegetable as well.

There are several cutting styles to choose from. Here is a partial listing.

1)	Round slices.	7)	Matchsticks.
2)	Diagonal slices.	8)	Shavings.
3)	Triangular shapes.	9)	Cubes, dicing and mincing.
4)	Rectangles.	10)	Wedge slices.
5)	Half-moons.	11)	Slicing cabbages.
6)	Quarters.	12)	Slicing big leafy greens.

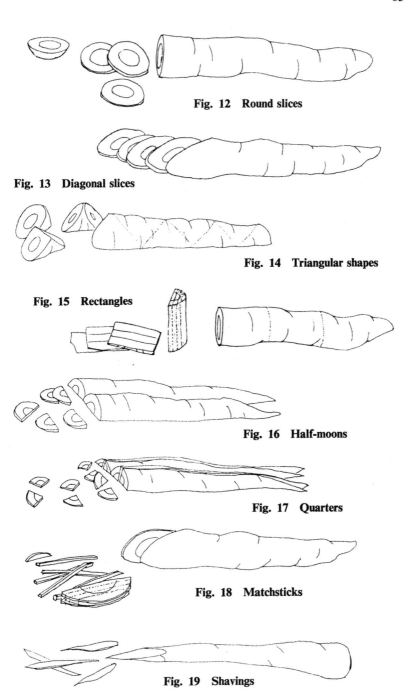

Fig. 12   Round slices

Fig. 13   Diagonal slices

Fig. 14   Triangular shapes

Fig. 15   Rectangles

Fig. 16   Half-moons

Fig. 17   Quarters

Fig. 18   Matchsticks

Fig. 19   Shavings

84

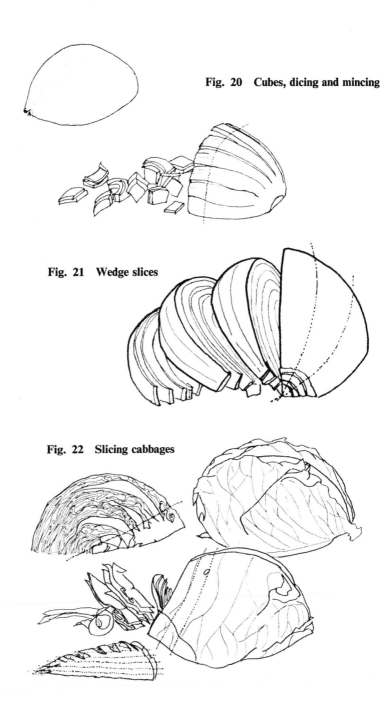

Fig. 20   Cubes, dicing and mincing

Fig. 21   Wedge slices

Fig. 22   Slicing cabbages

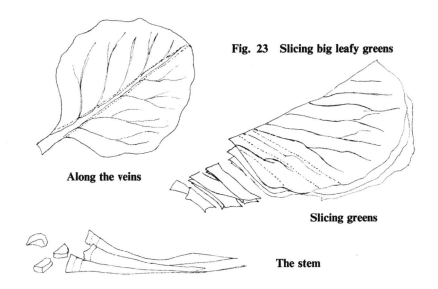

Fig. 23   Slicing big leafy greens

Along the veins

Slicing greens

The stem

Include a variety of different kinds of vegetables (roots, greens, ground and sea vegetables, for example) in a meal as well as an assortment of textures and colors. Also, use a variety of cooking styles. Here are some of the main methods that we use.

1. *Boiling methods:*   There are two main styles: quick, short time and slow, longer time boiling. You can have some kind of boiled vegetables at nearly every meal.

    A.   Quick boiling (blanching): The best way to cook your leafy green vegetables. Fill a pot with 1–2 inches of water which you bring to a rolling boil. Dip in your vegetables and take them out quickly. An oil skimmer lifts them up very easily. Drain the vegetables in This is perfect for cooking your green vegetables especially.

    The main point in this style is to cook in as short a time as possible, retaining crispness and bright colors. For example, watercress can be taken out after 15–30 seconds. Others take a little longer, in varying degrees, but not that much more. Kale, mustard greens, collard greens, cabbage, chinese cabbage, broccoli, cauliflower, celery and others can be used.

    A pinch of salt in the water helps to retain bright colors (but leave it out for bitter vegetables such as watercress and mustard greens as then the bitterness stays inside as well).

You can also cook root vegetables in this way but you have to cut them into very thin slices. You can boil them for a slightly longer time than you would with greens.

If you want to boil several different vegetables, do them one by one. Start with the lighter tasting varieties like the cabbages and end with more strong tasting ones like mustard greens so that the flavor of the latter won't effect the flavor of the former. Each vegetable's distinct individuality should be maintained.

You can use the leftover boiling water as a base for a soup. Or you can add some *kuzu* to it (2 teaspoons for 1 cup water) to thicken it into a sauce to pour over your vegetables. To do this: first dilute the *kuzu* in a small amount of water. Turn the flame to low underneath the boiled water and pour the *kuzu* in. Stir and simmer until the liquid turns clear. Add a little *tamari* soy sauce or *umeboshi* paste to taste and pour this over your boiled vegetables.

Boiled Chinese Cabbage and Watercress

Chinese cabbage leaves separated from the body but left whole
Uncut watercress
4 cups spring water

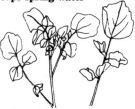

Fig. 23   Watercress

Put cabbage leaves into a pot of boiling water for 2–3 minutes. Take them out, and let them drain in a colander. Put watercress in the boiling water for a half a minute and drain them also. Pile three leaves at a time of Chinese cabbage on top of each other and cut them into 1″–2″ slices. Arrange them onto a serving plate. Add the watercress, making a decorative design and serve.

Boiled Salad

Chinese cabbage cut into 1″ slices
1 bunch of watercress
Carrots cut into matchsticks
4 cups spring water
Roasted sesame seeds

Quickly and separately boil the Chinese cabbage, carrots, and watercress (only until it turns a bright green). Drain each of them and mix them together into a serving bowl. Sprinkle the roasted sesame seeds on top.

B. Slow, longer time boiling: This style is basically for root vegetables such as *daikon*, carrots, onions, lotus root, burdock and so on, as well as squash. This style gives a calming but strong and healing energy.

One or two pieces of *kombu* are usually placed in the bottom of the pot to help prevent the vegetables from burning, to add extra minerals and flavor, and to help harmonize all the ingredients together.

The vegetables are then layered on top of the *kombu*, with the more yin ones on the bottom and the more yang ones on the top. The yin rising energy meets the yang descending energy and the dish is better integrated.

If the vegetables are fairly dry, put in enough water to just cover them. If they are fresh and more watery, cover them with water only halfway. Add a pinch of salt, cover the pot, bring everything up to a boil, turn the flame to low and simmer for about 20 minutes or until soft. The time depends on the type, quality and slice sizes of the vegetables used. Don't mix or stir the vegetables. When the vegetables are soft, add some *tamari* soy sauce for more flavor and simmer another 5 minutes. *Shiitake* mushrooms, dried *tofu*, *tempeh* and *seitan* may also be added to this dish.

Daikon, Lotus Root and *Shiitake* Mushrooms

1 *daikon*, sliced into ³⁄₄" rounds
1 lotus root, sliced into ¹⁄₄" rounds
3 *shiitake* mushrooms
1 piece *kombu*
1 pinch sea salt
Enough water to just cover
    the vegetables
Tamari soy sauce to taste

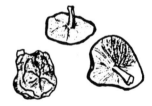

Fig. 24 *Shiitake* Mushroom

Place *kombu* in the bottom of the pot. Add the other ingredients in this order from the bottom up, *shiitake*, *daikon* and lotus root. Add water and sea salt, cover, and follow the above directions. Serves 3.

Dried *Daikon* and *Kombu*

1 cup dried *daikon* soaked until soft (10 minutes)
1 piece *kombu* 4"–5", washed & soaked 10 minutes

Enough water to just cover them
Tamari **soy sauce to taste**

Cut the *kombu* into thin, lengthwise, matchstick-like strips. Put it
into a pot and place the *daikon* on top. (Dried *daikon* comes in
shredded strips and can be found in natural food stores.) Add
enough water to just cover the *daikon*. You can use the soaking
water but if the *daikon* is too dark, discard its water. Add fresh
water if you don't have enough. Cover the pot, bring it to a boil,
lower the flame and simmer for 30–40 minutes until the *kombu*
becomes soft. Add *tamari* soy sauce to taste, boil away the excess
liquid and serve. Serves 2–3.

2. *Nishime style:* This is a very medicinal form of cooking using a
minimal amount of water. For this you need a heavy pot with a heavy
lid or some cookware specifically designed for waterless cooking.

   Kombu at the bottom of the pot helps to prevent burning as well as
adding extra minerals and taste.

   Root vegetables such as carrots, *daikon*, turnips, burdock, lotus root,
onions and hard winter squash (acorn, buttercup or Hokkaido), cabbage and *shiitake* mushrooms are normally used. They are usually cut
into 2″ chunks (except for burdock which is cut about half the size or
smaller) and layered on top of the *kombu* from yin to yang (yin on the
bottom). Squash dissolves and loses its shape if cooked for a long
time, so you may add it a little later on.

   To cook, soak a piece of *kombu* until it's soft, cut it into 1″ squares
and place it in the bottom of a pot. Add enough water just to cover
the *kombu* if the vegetables are fresh and watery. If they are dry or if
lotus root or burdock is used, add enough water to cover halfway.
Put in the vegetables and sprinkle a small amount of sea salt or *tamari*
soy sauce over them.

   Cover, set the flame on high until a steam is produced. Then lower
the flame and let the vegetables simmer peacefully for 15–20 minutes.
If water should evaporate during cooking, add a little more to the
bottom of the pot if it is necessary to prevent burning.

   When all the vegetables have softened, add a few more drops of
tamari to taste and mix the vegetables. You can do this by shaking
the pot up and down.

   Then, replace the cover and cook over a low flame for 2–5 minutes
more. After turning off the flame, remove the cover and let the vegetables sit for about 2 minutes. Serve the juice along with the vegetables
as it is very delicious.

Carrot, Lotus, Burdock *Nishime*

> 5 carrots, cut into 2″ chunks
> 3 lotus roots, cut into ¼″ chunks
> 2 burdock, cut into 1″ chunks
> 1 strip *kombu*, 6″–8″ long, soaked and sliced into 1″ pieces
> 2 pinches sea salt
> *Tamari* soy sauce to taste
> Enough water to cover vegetables halfway

Follow the above directions. Serves 6.

A few variation examples:

1) Carrots, cabbage, burdock, *kombu*
2) *Daikon, shiitake* mushrooms, *kombu*
3) Turnip, *shiitake* mushrooms, *kombu*
4) Carrots, lotus root, burdock, *kombu*
5) Onion, *kombu*
6) *Daikon*, lotus root, dried *tofu, kombu*
7) Parsnips, onions, *kombu*

Dandelion Roots/Dandelion Leaves

> Dandelion roots and leaves
> 1 tsp. dark sesame oil
> *Miso* or *tamari* soy sauce to taste

Wash and very finely slice the roots and leaves. Place the oil in a heated skillet and add the roots, cover and simmer with a high steam for 10 minutes or longer until they are soft. Add a few drops of water if needed to prevent burning. Then add the leaves, *miso* or *tamari* soy sauce to taste and simmer for another 2–4 minutes.

Other variations (finely chopped):

1) *Daikon* and its leaves or tops
2) Carrot and its tops (slice tops extra fine)
3) Radish and its tops
4) Dandelion root and leaves

3. *Sautéing:* There are two ways to sauté: with or without oil, using water as a substitute. When limiting your use of oil, you can use the water-sautéing method as often as you like.

It is best to use only sesame oil (particularly the dark or roasted variety) and to spread it onto the bottom of a heated pan rather than to pour it in. Put your oil into a cast-iron skillet (don't use too much, perhaps 1 tablespoon for 8 people) and heat it up with a medium high flame. To test if the oil is warm enough, drop in one slice of a vegetable. If the oil sizzles, then it is ready and you can put in the rest of the ingredients.

When "water sautéing," simply add a tablespoon or two of water as needed in cooking to prevent burning.

As an option, if using onions, many people like to sauté them first. I find that first sautéing them till they become translucent before putting in the next vegetable (move the onions on top of them) makes a very sweet dish.

Add the different kinds of vegetables one by one, starting with the ones that take the longest time to cook and ending with the faster cooking ones. For a more peaceful method, adjust the slices of the different vegetables so that they will cook at a uniform rate (thicker for softer ones and thinner for tougher ones) and layer them from yin to yang (yin on the bottom), cover and simmer without stirring.

Put in a pinch or two of sea salt from the beginning. Salt brings out the natural sweetness, draws out the water and helps to soften the vegetables quicker (it has the opposite effect on grains and beans and is therefore added later on in their case). Gently stir from time to time (with a wooden spoon or cooking chopsticks) to prevent burning.

After about 5 minutes you can turn the flame to low, cover (unless you are working with really watery items such as Chinese cabbage or *tofu*) and simmer until the vegetables are soft; the time it takes depends on what you're cooking and the size of your slices. You may need to add a little water to avoid burning, especially when cooking with something like burdock. Add a little *tamari* soy sauce (and some grated ginger if you wish) at the end for more flavor and simmer another 2–3 minutes. Uncover and boil away any excess water if there is any.

Any vegetable can be sautéed (cut your root vegetables into very thin slices or shavings) as can *tofu* and *tempeh*.

Two recipe examples:

Kinpira Carrots, Burdock

(This dish is very strengthening and can be used once or twice a week for those with more yin conditions such as asthma. When preparing this for persons who are avoiding oil, substitute with water and have it more often if you wish.)

1 cup shaved burdock
2 cups shaved carrots
Dark sesame oil (optional)
A pinch sea salt
Tamari soy sauce to taste

Optional: ½ tsp. grated ginger
Water, if needed to prevent burning
A few parsley sprigs

Heat oil or water in a skillet, sauté *tofu*, then celery and corn, adding a pinch of sea salt. Towards the end, add the radishes. Don't cover. Boil off any excess water. Add soy sauce to taste and simmer another 3 minutes. Add a dash of ginger and serve. Serves 3–4.

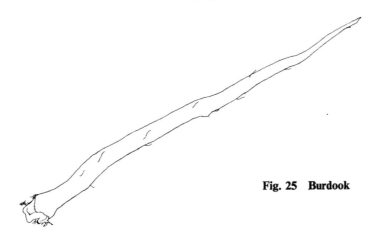

Fig. 25   Burdook

Chinese Cabbage
(This type of lighter dish using some of the "occasional use" vegetables is very nice for variety and freshness.

  3 Chinese cabbage leaves, sliced
  1 cup mung bean sprouts
  1 cake *tofu*
  8 snow peas
  Dark sesame oil or 1–2 Tbsps. water
  1 pinch sea salt
  Tamari soy sauce to taste
  A dash of grated ginger

Heat oil or water in a skillet, sauté *tofu*, cabbage and salt. Towards the end, add the snow peas and then the sprouts. Don't cover. Boil off any excess liquid. Add *tamari* soy sauce to taste and simmer another 3 minutes. Add a dash of ginger and serve. Serves 3–4.

4. *Pressure-cooking:* This is good for big chunks of root vegetables and squash (but don't cook greens this way). Use this style as often as you wish as long as you make sure that you are also making fresher vegetables such as salad and boiled or steamed greens to balance all the

pressure-cooking that you will be doing with your grains and beans. After the pressure comes up, carrots and onions may be done in 5 minutes and big chunks of lotus root and burdock in 15–20 minutes.

After putting your ingredients into the pressure-cooker, add enough water to just cover the bottom of the pot (maybe $\frac{1}{2}''$–$1''$). Add salt, cover, bring to pressure over a medium high flame. When up, turn the flame to low and simmer until done. Rinse the pot under cold water if you want to bring the pressure down quickly. (Don't uncover the pot until it's completely down.)

Lotus Root, *Daikon* and *Kombu*

> 2 lotus root, sliced into $\frac{1}{2}''$ rounds
> 2 *daikon*, sliced into 1" rounds
> 1 piece *kombu*
> 1 pinch sea salt
> $1\frac{1}{2}''$–2" water in the bottom of the pot

Put the *kombu* in the bottom of the pressure cooker and then add the *daikon*, lotus root, sea salt and water. Follow the above directions. Simmer for 20 minutes. Serves about 6.

Other variations:

1) Other root vegetables such as carrots, parsnips, onions, burdock and so on.
2) Buttercup or Hokkaido squash. (Use just enough water to cover the bottom of the pot. This is sweet and delicious.)
3) Add dried *tofu*, *seitan*, dried *daikon*, large round *fu* and/or *wakame*.

5. *Steaming:* You can use this method fairly often if you like. To steam, add $\frac{1}{2}''$–$1''$ of cold water in the bottom of a pot, insert a steamer, place your vegetable inside with a pinch of salt, cover, and bring the water to a boil. Then steam for 3–10 minutes or more until your vegetable is soft.

Good for any kind of vegetable and makes a nice variation to the boiled method. Be careful not to overcook them. Remove them while they're still crisp and brightly colored.

Steam each kind of vegetable separately unless you are going to serve them mixed together and they take the same amount of time to cook. When you put in a new vegetable, let the water cool a bit so that it gets cooked more evenly. If you want to keep their bright color, run the vegetables under cold water and don't cover them until they cool off. The leftover water can be used as soup stock or sauce (just like the boiling water). Steaming is a great way to heat up leftovers, especially rice.

Steamed Kale and Onions

    1 cup kale, cut into strips
    1 cup onions, thinly sliced
    1 pinch sea salt

Follow the above directions and steam for 5–10 minutes until soft.

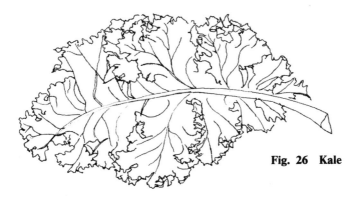

Fig. 26 Kale

6.   *Salad:*   There are three types of salads.

   A.   *Boiled salad:*   Refer to the section on boiled vegetables for directions and an example. This can be taken several times a week.

   B.   *Pressed salad:*   This can generally be eaten every two or three days. The vegetables are raw but pressing them with salt helps to yangize them. However, it may still be a little too yin for frequent use in cold weather for persons with severe diabetes. In this case, take this only once a week.

     To prepare, cut your vegetables into very, very thin slices or shred them and put them in a pickle press with sea salt for 45–60 minutes (or longer if you like). Drain off the excess water, wash off the excess salt and serve.

     If you don't have a pickle press you can put your vegetables in a bowl and cover them with a plate. Put a rock or some kind of weight (such as a large glass jar filled with water) on top of the plate and press.

Pressed Salad

    5 Chinese cabbage leaves, thinly sliced
    8 radishes, thinly sliced
    2 tsps. sea salt or 1 Tbsp. *umeboshi* juice.

Mix ingredients into a pickle press and follow the above directions. If too salty, quickly rinse in cold water before serving.

C. *Regular raw salad.* Persons trying to alleviate allergies should avoid this for a while, maybe a month or so. Otherwise, this is recommended about once or twice a week and more during the hot summer months.

You can use the usual vegetables such as lettuce, cucumbers, sprouts, carrots, onions, celery, parsley, etc., but avoid peppers, potatoes, tomatoes, eggplants and mushrooms. (You can also add roasted sesame and pumpkin seeds, wholewheat bread croutons, cooked chickpeas, pinto beans, rice, bulghur, couscous, noodles, macaroni, *wakame*, dried dulse and cooked *hijiki*, *arame*, *tofu*, *tempeh*, and *seitan*. Of course, your combinations have to be tasteful. Obviously, not all those ingredients are compatible with each other.)

Wakame Salad

- 1 cup *wakame* (Wash, soak 10 minutes, boil 2–3 minutes, rinse in cold water, drain & slice into 1″ pieces.)
- 1 iceberg lettuce cut into bite-size pieces
- 1 cucumber sliced into thin rounds.
- 1 Tbsp. *umeboshi* paste

Peel off the cucumber skin if it is waxed. Cut off the ends and with sea salt, rub them in a circular motion against the ends of the main body of the cucumber. This helps to draw out any bitterness if there is any. Rinse off the salt and slice. Mix with the *wakame*, lettuce and *umeboshi* paste. Serves 3.

Chickpea Salad

- ½ cup cooked chickpeas
- ½ cup cooked fresh corn kernels
- 1 onion, diced
- 1 cucumber, cut into little cubes
- 5 radishes, sliced

Mix all the ingredients together and add your preferred dressing (see *Dressing and Sauces* chapter).

7. *Baked:* This method takes a long time to cook but it gives strength and extra flavor. It's best to bake once in a while for variety rather than on a daily basis.

This style is good for squashes and root vegetables. You can leave them whole (burdock should be sliced) or cut them in half or in chunks.

You can bake them with or without oil, using a casserole dish or a cookie sheet covered with foil. If your vegetables are fresh and juicy you may not need to add water, especially if you oil the sheet or dish and have a good cover. If you don't use oil, add just a little water to cover the surface. If your vegetables are more dried out or are tough, add about a $\frac{1}{4}"-\frac{1}{2}"$ of water. Adding a dash of salt helps to draw out the water.

Place your vegetables, salt, water and/or oil into a dish or onto a sheet, cover, turn to 350°–375° F. and bake for 45–60 minutes, or until they're soft. Towards the end you can uncover, let any extra water (if any) evaporate, add *tamari* soy sauce, *miso* or some sauce to taste and simmer for another 5 minutes or so until done.

You can bake squash whole and uncovered on an oiled cookie sheet (with stuffing inside if you prefer). Or you can cut it in half and place the halves on the sheet (again uncovered) with the inside facing down. Don't forget to take out the seeds.

Baked Root Vegetables
1 lotus root, cut into $\frac{1}{2}"$ rounds
2 carrots, cut into triangular wedges
3 onions, quartered
1 burdock root, cut into diagonal slices
1 strip *kombu*
1 pinch sea salt
$\frac{3}{4}$ cup spring water

Place the *kombu* in the bottom of a casserole dish. Put all the vegetables on top of it, each in its own little corner of the dish. Add salt, water and cover. Bake at 350°–375° F. for 45–60 minutes or until soft. Uncover, add *tamari* soy sauce to taste, let some of the water evaporate, remove from the stove and serve. Serves about 4.

8. *Pickles:* Pickles are an extremely important addition to your diet. Have a small amount on the side at every meal or at least once a day and eat them with your grains. They aid in digestion, strengthen the flora in your intestines, stimulate your appetite and add zest to the meal.

Always use fresh, firm, and crisp vegetables for making pickles. Also, it is imperative that the vegetables, containers and anything else you use be thoroughly cleaned. You don't want any unknown substances interacting with the pickling process. For tougher vegetables, it is helpful to quickly blanch them in boiling water before pickling them.

Pickling time ranges from a couple of hours to several months. The main time factors are the size of your vegetables and the amount of salt you use. Small, thinly sliced pieces can be pickled very quickly where as large, thick or whole pieces take a long time. Long-time pickling requires more salt to retard the fermenting process. You can dip your vegetables in hot boiling water before you pickle them if you choose, especially with largely sliced and/or hard vegetables. This takes out the raw flavor and brings out a sweeter taste.

A lot of experimentation may be needed to get the feel of the right amount of salt to use. If the vegetables spoil before they pickle and/or not much water comes out (for methods that require that it does), then there isn't enough salt. If too much salt is added, the pickles will become too salty and any other flavor that the vegetables may have had will be covered up. To take out excess salt, rinse out or soak your pickles for a little while before you eat them.

If mold starts to form anywhere, remove it immediately so that the rest of the contents won't be affected.

Cover the whole thing with a cheesecloth. It helps to keep dirt and dust out of the pickles while letting the air circulate and enabling them to breathe. (Don't cover with an airtight lid.)

There are four main types of pickling methods that we usually use.

A. *Pressed pickles:* You can make them quickly, in a couple of hours, or you can make them in several weeks.

1) *Quick pickles:* When pickling for a few hours up to a day or two, you can use a pickle press. But since most of them are made out of plastic, it's not safe to use them for a longer period of time as the poisonous toxic substances in them will start to seep into the vegetables. If you don't have a press or if you want to use something safer, you can take a small glass bowl and find a saucer that fits into it. It should cover the inside as much as possible but still remain loose so that water can escape over the sides. For a weight, you can use a glass jar full of water, grains or beans or some clean stones.

Soft, watery vegetables like thinly sliced cucumbers and very thin matchstick *daikon* strips can be done in 2–3 hours. Other pickles can be made in the morning and be either eaten for dinner or left for 2–3 days longer. Some (like harder, less watery vegetables like turnips) may need the extra time. Again, it mostly depends on the size of the pieces.

The vegetables have to be cut into really thin slices or shredded for this method. (An exception is mustard greens which can be made whole and cut when you want to eat them. Mix the salt in well and wait 2–3 days.) Chinese cabbage, red and white cabbage, *daikon* and its greens, turnips and its greens, celery, radishes, onions, cucumbers and bok-choy are good to use. For best results, use only one kind of vegetable at a time. You can add a strip of *kombu* (perhaps 3″–6″ long for two cups of vegetables) for extra minerals and a different flavor. Soak the *kombu* until it's soft, slice it into thin strips and put it underneath the vegetables. Grated ginger can be added if you wish.

For 2 cups of vegetables add about 1–2 teaspoons of salt. Mix them together thoroughly. The salt can be substituted with 2–4 teaspoons of *umeboshi* vinegar, paste, or plums and/or *shiso* leaves. You can also use 2–4 tablespoons of *tamari* soy sauce. Water will start to rise above the saucer or pressure plate. If there is a lot you can take a little out but always leave some of it covering the plate. Cover with a cheesecloth (not necessary if using a press of course) and wait till it's all done.

Daikon Top Pickles

2 cups *daikon* tops (the greens), shredded
1 tsp. sea salt

Wash and slice the *daikon* tops into shreds. Then add the sea salt. Taste the greens. They should taste somewhat salty but it shouldn't be an overpowering saltiness. If it is, add more greens. If you can't taste the salt, add a little more of it. Press, following the above directions. Pickle for 6–8 hours or have them the next day.

2) *Longer time pressed pickles:* A wooden keg or ceramic crock are good containers to use for this. A heavy stone or large jar filled with water is placed on top of a plate or a wooden disc which fits inside for pressure. Cover the whole thing with a cheesecloth and place in a cool dark place. Check regularly for mold and remove it immediately if any appears. Sauerkraut is made this way. Below is a sample recipe.

Sauerkraut

5 lbs. cabbage, shredded
⅓ cup sea salt

Pickle following the above directions. If the water doesn't rise up to or above the plate within 10–20 hours, add more salt and/or add more weight. Keep in a cool, dark place and it should be done 1½–2 weeks later. Store the finished product in the refrigerator.

B.   *Brine pickles:*   To make this pickle, tightly stuff some vegetables into a glass jar. Boil some kind of a brine mixture, let it cool off and pour it into the jar, filling it up. Cover the top with cheesecloth which you can fasten down with a rubber band and pickle for several days. When done, store them in a refrigerator. This is how dill pickles are made. Beside cucumbers, you can use onions, turnips, rutabagas, *daikon*, carrots, broccoli, cauliflower, cabbages, greens and so on.

There are several kinds of brine that you can choose to use, examples of which I have presented below. You can use a soup stock if you want. You can add ginger, *kombu*, *shiitake* mushrooms, lemon juice and rinds, *shiso* leaves, grated raw apple and so on, for extra flavor. Some *ame* rice syrup can be boiled and dissolved into the brine (good with the *tamari* based one) for a sweet taste.

Cauliflower and/or Broccoli (Salt-Based Brine)

Enough cauliflower pieces to fill a quart jar
1 carrot, thinly sliced into half-moons
1 strip *kombu*, 3″–4″ long
2–3 cups spring water
¼ cup sea salt

Bring *kombu*, salt and water to a boil. Then turn off the flame and cool the liquid. Wash and place the cauliflower and carrots into a quart jar. Pour the cooled liquid over the vegetables into the jar. Cover with a cheesecloth and let sit 3–4 days till done. After they are done, store the pickles in the refrigerator.

Mustard Green Pickles (*Tamari*-Based Brine)

1 bunch mustard greens, washed & cut into 1″ slices
½ cup *tamari* soy sauce
½ cup spring water
2 tsps. *ame* rice syrup
2 Tbsps. sesame seeds, washed & dry-roasted
1 Tbsp. fresh grated ginger

Place the mustard greens and sesame seeds into a glass jar. Bring *tamari*, water and rice syrup to a boil. Turn off the flame and add the grated ginger to the liquid. Let the brine cool and then pour it into the jar over the greens and seeds. Cover the top of the jar with cheesecloth and let it sit one day. It is now ready to eat. Keep in the refrigerator. Turnip or *daikon* greens may also be used.

Lotus Root Pickles (*Umeboshi*-Based Brine)

3 lotus roots, sliced into very thin rounds
1 cup water
1 cup *umeboshi* vinegar
5 *shiso* leaves

Dip the lotus roots quickly in some boiling water and place them in a jar. Mix the water, *umeboshi* vinegar and *shiso* leaves together and pour everything into the jar. Cover with cheesecloth and let sit 3–4 days.

C. *Miso pickles:* *Miso* pickles are especially helpful for recovering good digestive strength. They are simple to make. Just quickly blanch your vegetables in boiling water and then submerge and surround them totally in *miso*. This is used for root vegetables such as carrots, burdock, *daikon*, turnips, parsnips and ginger. Broccoli stems make great pickles as well. Greens are too watery.

The vegetables have to be dried out until you can band them like rubber before you put them into the *miso*. Otherwise, the *miso* will get too watery and the pickling won't work.

Pickling time depends on the vegetables you use and the size of your slices. Very thin ones can pickle in 3–4 days, up to a week. Whole vegetables with slits in their sides can take 1–2 weeks, thick slices about 3 months and whole vegetables (unslitted) can be left in the *miso* up to a year. Just make sure they are totally submerged (top, bottom, and sides). You don't need to use any pressure.

When the pickles are done, just take them out, rinse them off, slice them and eat them.

Broccoli Stem *Miso* Pickles

Broccoli Stems
A container of *miso*

Take your leftover broccoli stems. Peel them unless the skins are soft, quickly blanch them in boiling water and submerge them into the *miso* for 1–2 weeks, depending on how thick they are. You can leave the skins on if you like. The pickling time will be much longer then, maybe a month or more. Cover with a cheesecloth and keep in a cool, dark place until they are done.

D. *Bran pickles:* This involves pickling in a mixture of bran (rice or wheat) or rice flour, and sea salt. Like *miso* pickles, bran pickles are especially good for weak intestines.

Quickly dry-roast the bran or flour in a skillet over a medium low flame until a nutty fragrance is emitted. Remove from the skillet and allow it to cool.

Firm, root vegetables pickle best but you can also use greens. The vegetables should all be dried before you use them. A few hours under the sun would be great. *Daikon*, carrots and parsnips are best when dried longer (several days), until they bend like rubber.

A ceramic crock or wooden keg again are the best containers to use. Cover the pickles with a cheesecloth and keep the container in a cool, dark place.

There are two ways to make bran pickles.

1) *Bran pickles ♯1:* Boil some salt and water, let that cool off, place in a crock or keg and thoroughly mix in the roasted bran or flour to form a paste. Take your dried vegetables and totally submerge them into this paste making sure that the vegetables aren't touching each other. Pack this whole thing down until it's firm and solid. Cover with a cheesecloth.

If you slice the vegies into fairly small pieces they will be done in a week or two. You can also leave them whole. Whole root vegetables can take as long as 3–5 months to pickle. Add more salt if you want to pickle for a long time. (Whole leaves take only a couple of weeks.)

As you remove your finished pickles, you can keep adding new vegetables. When you do that, add more bran and salt. Mix the paste once in a while. If kept well, you can use this paste for years as you add and subtract vegetables from it.

Short Time Paste Proportions (1–2 Weeks)

    10–12 cups bran or rice flour
    ⅛–¼ cup sea salt
    3–5 cups water

Longer Time Paste Proportions (Up to 3–5 Months)

    10–12 cups bran or rice flour
    1½–2 cups sea salt
    3–5 cups water

2) *Bran pickles ♯2:* This method is made by alternating layers of vegetables with layers of the bran and sea salt mixture.

Mix roasted bran with sea salt and cover the bottom of a crock or keg. Then, add a layer of dried vegetables. Add another layer of bran and salt. Keep alternating. The last layer should be bran. Insert a plate or a wooden disc into the crock on top of the mixture, place a heavy weight on top and press the whole thing. The plate or disc should fit inside the container. It should be loose fitting but cover the contents as much as possible. A clean stone or a jar filled with water can be used as a weight. Cover with a cheesecloth and put in a cool, dark place. When water begins to rise, lighten the weight. When pickles are done, rinse off the bran, slice and eat.

Just as in *Bran pickles #1*, you can either slice the vegies into fairly small pieces or leave them whole. As before, whole pieces take a much longer time to pickle and require more salt.

● *Short Time Proportions (1–2 Weeks)*

10–12 cups bran or rice flour
⅛–¼ cup sea salt

● *Longer Time Proportions (3–5 Months)*

10–12 cups bran or rice flour
2–3 cups sea salt

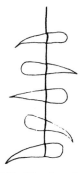

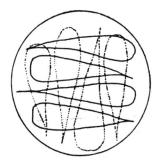

Fig. 27 Hanging *daikon* to dry   **Fig. 28 Layering *daikon* in a keg**

Daikon Bran Pickles (*Takuan*)

10 *daikon* radishes
Bran & salt using longer time proportions

Dry the *daikon* for a few days until you can bend them like rubber into a semi-circle. A good way to dry them is to string several *daikons* together with a strong string and let them hang for a few days. When you tie the *daikon*, leave enough string length between each one so that they don't touch each other.

Dry-roast the salt in a skillet until it becomes shiny. Remove salt, then quickly dry-roast the bran until it emits a nutty fragrance. Stir constantly to prevent it from burning. Remove and mix bran and salt together.

Sprinkle and evenly spread a handful of the bran/salt mixture into the bottom of a wooden keg or ceramic crock. Place several *daikon* inside, laying them side by side but not touching each other (otherwise they may spoil). Totally cover with a layer of bran and salt.

Add another layer of *daikon*, this time placing them side by side at right angles from the previous layer. Cover with bran/salt and continue alternating. If you have any *daikon* leaves, make a layer of those on top. Top everything off with a final layer of bran/salt.

Place a flat wooden disc or plate inside the crock with a heavy weight on top. Cover the whole thing with cheesecloth.

Pickle for a year. This is best when made at the end of the summer and taken out a year later in the fall. The leaves on top may be taken out in a month or two.

Variations:

1) Quicker *daikon* pickles. Dry *daikon* under the sun for one day only. Cut them in half lengthwise. Layer as above (using long time bran/salt proportions), place a 20–30 pound weight on top and cover with a cheesecloth. A few days later, when water rises to the top, lighten the weight to 5–10 pounds. Take the *daikon* out in two weeks.

2) Chinese cabbage bran pickles. Take two heads of Chinese cabbage. Separate and dry the leaves in the sun for two days. Layer as above with short time bran/salt proportions and place a weight and cheesecloth on top. In about 10 hours water should rise to the top (if not, add more weight and/or salt). Remove all the water, relayer the leaves with bran/salt, add a weight, cover with cloth and it should be ready in a week.

11. Beans and Bean products ▬▬▬▬▬▬▬

Most helpful dishes include:

Azuki beans or lentils cooked with sea vegetables or root and round vegetables
Dried _tofu_ with sea vegetables and vegetables

Beans are high in protein and are a delicious addition to your diet. It is important not to overeat beans, to chew them very well, and to cook them thoroughly, otherwise you can have gas, intestinal problems and a sluggish condition. They should always be a side dish, not compromising more than 15% of the meal. As they make a heavier dish, beans are more appropriate for supper, somewhat less often for lunch and generally not for breakfast.

Azuki beans, chickpeas, lentils and black soybeans are the most yang beans and the best ones to use on a regular basis. Use these beans and/or bean products such as _tofu_ and _tempeh_ about three to six times a week (but in small quantities) when healing. Other beans such as pintos, kidneys, black beans and red lentils can be eaten occasionally, about once a week or less during the healing process or may be avoided altogether for several months. Soybeans (which are full of protein) need particular attention so that they are cooked thoroughly. They are delicious in combination with vegetables. They can also be eaten in the form of _tofu_, _tempeh_, _natto_, _miso_ and _tamari_ soy sauce.

Store beans in an airtight container, like a glass jar, in a cool dry place.

When washing beans, first spread them out a little at a time and take out any stones or anything else that may be mixed in. Then place the beans in a bowl and submerge them in water and stir. Rinse off any dust that may rise to the surface. Repeat this about 3 times or until the water becomes clear. As you lift the beans out of the water into a strainer or colander to drain, leave out any heavy dust or residue that may remain in the bottom of the bowl.

Except for red and green lentils, beans may be soaked for a few hours or overnight prior to cooking. This softens them and helps to cook them quicker. _Azuki_ beans need only a few hours of soaking and from time to time you may cook them without it, particularly when trying to strengthen an overly yin condition. Soaking is preferred for pinto and kidney beans for more digestibility. Chickpeas and soybeans need it no matter what, as they are so tough. Use the soaking water when cooking.

Salt is to be added towards the end of the cooking process after the beans have already softened, otherwise they will remain hard for a long time. Placing a piece of *kombu* on the bottom of the pot also helps to soften them as well as adding more minerals and flavor. There are three main ways to cook beans.

1. *Boiling:* This is the method I prefer the most as it cooks the beans gently, slowly, thoroughly and they turn out really delicious and much sweeter.

   Soak the beans for a few hours or overnight (not necessary for lentils and split peas). Place an optional piece of *kombu* on the bottom, then your choice of optional vegetables and finally the beans on top. Add just enough water to cover the beans a little bit. Place a drop top inside the pot so that it sits directly over the beans. This top should be loose fitting to let steam escape on the sides but large enough to cover the inside as much as possible.

   As the beans expand, slowly and gently pour more *cold* water down the sides of the pot from time to time, always enough to just cover them. The sudden cold water helps the beans soften more quickly. Bring this to a boil over a medium flame.

   Then, turn the flame to medium low and let it simmer for 45 minutes to an hour or so, continuing to add cold water once in a while. Watch closely to see when more water is needed to prevent burning. Don't stir or mix at all, letting the cooking go on undisturbed. This makes for a tastier dish.

   When the beans are 70% done, add salt and/or *miso* or *tamari* soy sauce, remove the drop top, and simmer for another 10–20 minutes or so until the beans are completely soft, boiling away any excess liquid.

Azuki Beans, Squash and *Kombu*
(Gives vitality, strengthens spleen, pancreas, stomach, and digestion.)

1 cup *azuki* beans
2 cups buttercup or Hokkaido squash
1 piece *kombu*, 3″–6″ long
Spring water, added little by little
$\frac{1}{2}$–1 tsp. sea salt
***Optional: miso* or *tamari* soy sauce to taste**
Drop top

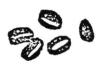
Fig. 29   *Azuki* beans

Place *kombu* in a pot. Then, cut the squash into big chunks and place them inside followed by the beans and water. Follow the above directions. This dish can also be pressure-cooked. When squash is not in season, you may use carrots, turnips, rutabagas, parsnips or onions. Also, the *azuki* beans may be substituted with lentils or other beans. Serves 6.

2. *Pressure-cooking:* This is the best method for chickpeas as they are extremely hard and tough. *Azuki,* pinto and kidney beans can also be pressure-cooked.

   Red and green lentils, split peas and black and white soybeans may clog the pressure gauge of the pressure cooker and cause a possible explosion, so it is best to boil them. In the case of the lentils and split peas it doesn't matter much as they soften very quickly anyway. With soybeans, there are three things you can do to make them safer for pressure-cooking.

   A. Boil the (presoaked) soybeans and skim off all the foam that rises to the top. When no more foam appears (maybe in a half hour), place them in a pressure-cooker and cook till done.
   B. Dry-roast the soybeans before pressure-cooking them. Combining black soybeans with rice or another grain in addition to the roasting, helps even further.
   C. Soak black soybeans for several hours or overnight with ⅛ tsp. of sea salt for every cup of beans. This helps to prevent the skins from coming off and clogging the gauge.

Chickpeas

> **2 cups chickpeas soaked overnight**
> **½ cup onions, diced**
> **¼ cup carrots, diced**
> **¼ cup burdock, diced**
> **1 strip *kombu*, 3″–6″ long**
> **5–6 cups spring water**
> **½ tsp. sea salt**
> ***Tamari* soy sauce to taste**

Layer the ingredients in this order; first *kombu*, then onions, carrots, burdock and finally chickpeas. Add the water and pressure-cook for 60–75 minutes. Turn the flame off and let the pressure come down. Then, take off the cover, add salt and *tamari* soy sauce to taste and continue cooking until most of the liquid has boiled away. Mix and serve. Serves 6–8.

3. *Baking:* This is delicious in the winter as it is very hearty. This method takes the longest time to prepare but the results are well worth the wait. Pintos, kidneys and soybeans yield well to baking.

To prepare, first place the pre-soaked beans in a pot on top of the stove, adding 4–5 cups of water for every cup of beans. Bring this to a boil, and boil for 15–20 minutes to loosen the bean skins.

Then, pour this whole thing into a baking pot. (You can place an optional piece of *kombu* underneath.) Cover, place in the oven and bake at 350 degrees F., adding more water from time to time as the beans need it. They may be done in about 3–4 hours depending on the beans you use.

You may add some vegetables halfway through. The salt and/or *tamari* soy sauce or *miso* should be added after the beans have become soft and creamy. After adding the salt, you can take the cover off and let the beans brown a bit. Then remove from the stove and serve.

Baked Pinto Beans (Kidneys may be substituted)

2 cups pinto beans, soaked
1 cup fresh corn kernels
½ cup onions
½ cup carrots
2 pinches sea salt
8 cups spring water
1 piece *kombu*, 3″–6″ long

Bake following the above directions.

Other bean variations (pressure-cooking or boiling preferable:)

1) *Azuki* with carrots and onions
2) *Azuki* with chestnuts
3) *Azuki* with parsnips
4) *Azuki* with raisins and/or rice syrup

Bean Products:

While you are healing, it is best not to over consume bean products. Have a small amount 2–3 times a week.

1. *Tofu* or soybean curd comes in two forms, fresh and dried. The fresh *tofu* available in Oriental shops is usually prepared using a modern, chemicalized curdling agent and it is best to buy natural *tofu* curdled with *nigari* (which comes from sea salt). This is available in natural food stores. Dried *tofu* is more strengthening and can be used regularly by anyone. Fresh *tofu* is more yin and should be cooked, especially with some sea vegetables, for persons who are recovering from allergies.

    a) *Fresh tofu:* When you buy fresh *tofu*, open the package and store the *tofu* in the refrigerator submerged in fresh water (throw out the water it came in). Before you cook with it, very quickly rinse it under the tap.

. *Tofu* cooks very quickly and can be boiled, steamed, baked or broiled, sautéed or pan-fried. It's actually done as soon as it's heated up. It can be prepared in many ways.

When boiling *tofu*, cut it into cubes, put it into boiling water and when it rises to the top it is finished. Add it to soup towards the end of preparation. For *miso* soup, put in the *tofu* just before you add the *miso*.

To steam *tofu*, cut it into smaller cubes and steam until it becomes hot.

When sautéing with *tofu*, you don't need to add any extra water as a lot of it will come out of the *tofu*. You can press out the excess liquid. To do this, place the whole cube onto a wooden cutting board and prop the board up on one end. Put another cutting board, a heavy plate or a weight on top of the *tofu* and let it drain for one hour.

When pan-frying, baking or broiling, cut the *tofu* into slabs, heat a thin layer of oil or water in a skillet or baking/broiling sheet, add the *tofu* and cook the slices till they brown and/or become hot. This only takes a few minutes so be careful not to burn them. Before or after cooking you may spread, dip or marinate each slice in one of several sauces or dips including: 1) grated ginger and *tamari* soy sauce, 2) dry-roasted sesame seeds with *tamari* soy sauce, 3) diluted *miso* and chopped onions or scallions.

Boiled *Tofu*, Chinese Cabbage and Carrots

1 cube of *tofu*
3–5 Chinese cabbage leaves cut into 1″ slices
1 carrot cut into very thin slices
2–3 cups spring water
1 piece *kombu* 3″–6″ long
1 Tbsp. *tamari* soy sauce
2–3 chopped scallions
1 tsp. grated ginger

Make a *kombu* stock by boiling, then simmering the *kombu* and water for 2–3 minutes. Place the carrots, Chinese cabbage and *tofu* into separate sections of the pot and boil them for a few minutes until they are done. Make a dip by taking 1 tablespoon of the stock and mixing in the *tamari*, scallions and ginger. Serves 2–3.

b) *Dried tofu:* You can buy dried *tofu*. They look like thin, lightly yellow, rectangular wafers. To cook with it, first soak it in water until it softens. Then cut it up into any desired size or leave it whole. This can then be combined with vegetables and treated like one of them. It should be boiled at least 15 minutes. You can also pressure-cook it and add it to soups and stews. Below is a recipe example.

Hijiki (or *Arame*) with Onions, Carrots and Dried *Tofu* (Sautéed)

1 cup *hijiki* (or *arame*), soaked
½ cup onions, thin half-moon slices
½ cup carrots, thin matchstick
½ cup dried *tofu*, soaked & cut into matchsticks
A few drops of dark sesame oil or water
Soaking water
1 Tbsp. *tamari* soy sauce

Put oil or water into a skillet and heat it up. Sauté the onions until they are translucent, add and sauté the carrots and finally add and sauté the sea vegetable. Put in the *tofu*, add water until it's level with the ingredients, cover, simmer for 15–20 minutes or until everything is soft. Then add *tamari* soy sauce to taste, uncover, boil away excess liquid and serve. Serves 6.

3. *Tempeh:* This is a fermented soy product used in Indonesia and now available in many natural food stores. It's energizing and full of protein. Store it in the refrigerator.

Note: Since *tempeh* is innoculated with a fungus spore in its processing, it may initially cause a reaction for some allergic people.

You can cook *tempeh* anywhere from a few minutes to 30 minutes or more. The longer that you cook it the more easily digestible and smoother tasting it becomes.

In boiling, steaming, pressure-cooking, baking and sautéing with vegetables, if the *tempeh* is pan- or deep-fried beforehand it makes the dish extra delicious. It can be deep-fried without any batter or covering. Unlike fresh *tofu*, add it to your dishes in the beginning of the cooking preparation.

Tempeh and *Arame*

1 *tempeh*, sliced into small cubes
1 cup *arame*, soaked (see *Sea Vegetable* chapter)
2 onions, sliced into thin half-moons

1 cup water, including soaking water
1 pinch sea salt
Tamari **soy sauce to taste**
Several parsley sprigs

Place onions, followed by *arame* and then *tempeh* in a small pan or

4. *Natto:*   This is an odd stringy, fermented soybean preparation. To
    some individuals at the first encounter, it is also unpleasant smelling.
    But once a taste is acquired for *natto*, many people can't get enough
    of it.

    This is not an absolutely necessary food such as rice, sea vegetables,
    greens, root vegetables, *miso*, and so on, so have it only if you want
    some. It is protein-rich like all the other soy products and good for
    vitality as well as being very easy to assimilate. You can find this in
    natural or Oriental food stores.

    It usually comes frozen, so you have to thaw it out by leaving it for
    a day in the refrigerator compartment (out of the freezer) or a few
    hours in room temperature. Otherwise, store it in the freezer until the
    day you want to eat it.

    Stir in one or more of the following ingredients: 1) grated *daikon*,
    2) grated ginger, 3) chopped scallions or 4) diced raw onions with the
    addition of either 1) *tamari* soy sauce, 2) *umeboshi* paste or 3) sauer-
    kraut. Pieces of *nori* may also be mixed in. These combinations may be
    eaten on top of your rice or other grains as a condiment or in *miso*
    soup.

12. Sea Vegetables ▬▬▬▬▬▬▬▬

Sea vegetables are a very important and integral part of the macrobiotic diet. They help purify and strengthen the bloodstream and strengthen the intestines, digestive system, liver, pancreas, sexual organs, and mental clarity and awareness. They also help promote beautiful skin and hair. They can be consumed everyday in some form no matter what your condition. They supply calcium, iron, protein, iodine, and vitamins A, B_{12}, and C as well as various other minerals.

Many people used to (and some still do) cringe at the thought of eating sea vegetables and considered it an esoteric Oriental food. However, they have been consumed traditionally by people all over the world including the Celtics, Vikings, Russians, coastal Africans, Mediterranean peoples, North and South American Indians, native Australians, and the early New England settlers (dulse and *kombu* in their case) as well as in the Far East. Some varieties may take a while to acquire a taste for but it is well worth the effort for all the countless benefits that they bestow.

Sea vegetables are purchased dried (from natural food stores) and can therefore last many years until you use them. They are also easily stored. Any shady, dry place will do.

There are several varieties that are now available. *Kombu* is more tough and may take several hours, unless pressure-cooked, to completely soften. Dulse, on the other hand, can be eaten raw or like *nori*, just toasted for a second.

Wash sea vegetables very quickly to retain as much of their nutrients as possible. Submerge *hijiki, wakame* and *arame* in water, rinse off any dust that floats to the top and lift them out of the water, leaving any sand or stones that sit at the bottom. (*Arame* will probably be pretty clean already as it has been shredded.)

To clean *kombu*, brush off any dirt or dust with a dry or wet towel. Leave the white colored substance (which consist of salt and complex sugars) on the surface of the *kombu* as they contribute to its flavor and value. Dulse doesn't need to be washed in water but check it very carefully for hidden shells, stones, and tiny fish. *Nori* and agar-agar shouldn't be washed.

1. *Arame and hijiki:*   *Arame* comes shredded and has a very delicious but mild flavor. *Hijiki* is naturally stringy and looks like a thicker, darker *arame*. It also has a richer taste. *Hijiki* should be soaked for 3–5 minutes beforehand until it expands a bit. Remember that it finally become 3–5 times larger so be careful not to use more than

you need. It isn't necessary to soak *arame*, just *quickly* rinse it once in cold water.

Arame and *hijiki* are cooked the same ways, though *hijiki* takes a longer time, and one can be substituted for the other. They combine really well with root vegetables or with *seitan, tofu, tempeh,* and fresh corn as well as other ingredients. They are generally sautéed or just simmered with a small amount of water.

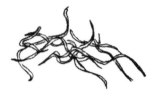

Fig. 30   Dried *arame*   Fig. 31   Dried *hijiki*

Hijiki (or _Arame_), Lotus Root, Leeks and _Shiitake_ Mushrooms

> **1 cup _hijiki_ (or _arame_), soaked**
> **1 lotus root, cut into very thin rounds**
> **1 leek, cut into $\frac{1}{4}$" slices**
> **2 _shiitake_ mushrooms, soaked & thinly sliced**
> **$\frac{1}{2}$ Tbsp. dark sesame oil or water**
> **Soaking water**
> **1–2 Tbsps. _tamari_ soy sauce**

Soak *hijiki* (or *arame*) until you can slice easily. Place all the sea vegetable onto a cutting board and cut through it, with the slices being 3" apart from each other. Then cut some more 3" slices at right angles to the previous ones.

Add oil or water to a skillet and heat it up. Layer the *hijiki*, then the *shiitake*, lotus root and finally the leeks. Add water until it is level with the vegetables. Cover and let this simmer over a medium low flame until everything is soft. Then uncover, add the *tamari* soy sauce and simmer another 5–10 minutes or more, boiling away any remaining liquid. Serves 4–5.

2. *Kombu:*   This comes in thick, flat strips which may be anywhere from 3"–18" long. There are recipes throughout this cookbook using *kombu* as it enhances the flavor of grains, beans and vegetable dishes, helping them to soften and/or effectively combining and synthesizing all the ingredients into a whole. It also makes an excellent soup stock. (See *Soup* chapter.) In all of those cases, the *kombu* is more like an acces-

sory but you can also use it as a vegetable in its own right. It has a pretty tough texture, so a pressure-cooker really comes in handy though you can also boil it for a while.

Before you can slice it, you need to soak it. It doubles in size when you do. Soak only until it is soft enough to cut. Otherwise, it becomes very slippery and slicing will become difficult.

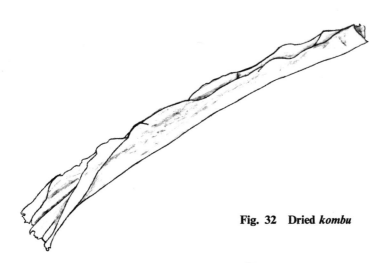

Fig. 32 Dried *kombu*

Pressure-cooked *Kombu* and Carrots

12″ strip *kombu*, soaked & sliced into 1″ squares
5 carrots, cut into triangular wedges
Soaking water
1 Tbsp. *tamari* soy sauce

Clean, soak, and slice *kombu* and place in the bottom of a pressure cooker. Add carrots, *tamari* and water to half cover the vegetables. Cover, bring to pressure, turn the flame to low and simmer 15–20 minutes. You may uncover and boil away the excess water to make a sweeter dish. Serves 6.

Lotus Seeds and *Kombu*
(This dish is especially helpful for respiratory problems, asthma and hay fever.)

½ cup lotus seeds
6″ strip *kombu*
A few drops of *tamari* **soy sauce**

Soak lotus seeds with *kombu* for 6–8 hours or overnight. Slice the *kombu* into 1″ slices. Then place the *kombu* and seeds into a pot with enough water to just cover them, cover, bring to a boil, turn flame to low and simmer until they become soft. Add a few drops of *tamari* to taste and simmer another 3–5 minutes. (You may also use dried or fresh lotus root instead of the seeds.) Serves 4.

3. *Wakame:* This is a thin, leafy type of sea vegetable and cooks quickly. You can use it in any recipe that calls for *kombu*. As is *kombu*, it is excellent in grain, bean, vegetable dishes and soups.

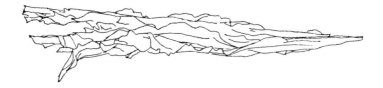

Fig. 33   Dried *wakame*

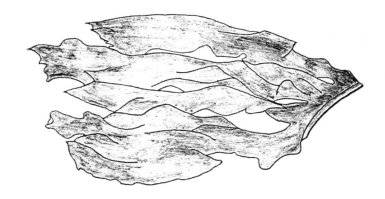

Fig. 34   Soaked *wakame*

Wakame should also be soaked before you can slice it. If the soaking water is a bit salty, you can save it for soups, grains or bean dishes, where it will be more diluted. Or if you want to use some of the flavor that went into the liquid for your *wakame* dish, combine a portion of it with fresh water.

The vein portion takes a longer time to cook so slice that part fairly thinly so that it will be finished when the softer leafy sections (which should be sliced into larger pieces) are.

(Look under *Vegetables, Soups* and *Condiments* for more *wakame* recipes.)

Wakame and *Ginger*
(Good for dissolving excess oils and animal fats.)

2 cups *wakame*, washed, soaked and sliced
1 tsp. ginger, freshly grated
Spring water
***Tamari* soy sauce**

Slice the harder vein of the *wakame* into smaller pieces than the soft leafy portion. Quickly blanch the sea vegetable in some boiling water. Remove, drain the *wakame* in a colander and save the water for soups or other dishes. Place the sea vegetable into individual serving dishes and add ¼ teaspoon of grated ginger on top with a drop of *tamari* soy sauce. For variety, boil together with greens or finely chopped root vegetables. Serves about 6.

4. *Nori:* This comes in thin, flat, paper-like sheets. No washing, soaking and cooking is required except to lightly toast it over an open flame for a few seconds. In Japan it is used to garnish noodles, grains, and vegetables as well as acting as wrapping for *sushi* and rice balls among other things.

After toasting the sheets, you can leave them whole (as you would when you make *sushi* rolls) or cut them up with your fingers or scissors into any size pieces that you desire. Very small pieces or slivers make a good decorative garnish on top of noodles, grains, vegetables, and so on. One eighth of a sheet is a nice size for covering and picking up small pieces of grains or vegetables. Two pieces (a quarter of a sheet each) are used to wrap a rice ball.

Norimaki (*Sushi*)
(They are handy as appetizers, snacks and for traveling and have a very decorative appearance.)

1 ½ cups cooked short-grain (sticks best) brown rice
1 sheet *nori*
1 carrot cut into several lengthwise strips
2–3 uncut (except for the roots) scallions
1″ boiling water in a pot
¼–½ tsp. *umeboshi* paste
1 pinch sea salt

Add a pinch of salt (for brighter vegetable colors) to the pot of boiling water and boil the carrot strips until they are soft. Take the strips out and let them drain. Then, boil the scallions (cut off the roots) for just a second or before they loose the bright green color, take them out and let them drain as well.

Meanwhile, toast a sheet of *nori* by passing it several times over an open flame (on the dull side only for easier rolling) until it's green but not so much that it is overly crisp and crinkly.

Place a *sushi* mat onto a cutting board and the sheet of *nori* on top of it. The halfway fold of the *nori* should be horizontal from you. Wet your hands and evenly press ¼″ layer of rice onto the *nori*, leaving ½″–¾″ of the top edge (the side away from you) and ¼″ of the bottom edge uncovered. Then, make a horizontal indentation in the rice 1″ up from the bottom of the *nori* and spread the *umeboshi* paste inside the length of it. Then press 1–3 carrot strips and the scallions (again horizontally) on top of the paste.

Next, slowly roll the mat and it's contents upwards, pressing firmly upon the rice and other ingredients. Try to tuck the vegetables underneath as you keep rolling. Wet the top edge of the uncovered *nori* (to help in sealing) and complete the roll.

Wash and dry your hands. Place the roll with the sealed edge underneath, wet a vegetable knife (to prevent the rice from sticking to it for smooth, easy cutting), and slowly, carefully but firmly cut the roll into 1″ slices. Place the slices onto a plate with the inside turned upwards to show it's beautiful design, decorate and serve. Serves 5 pieces.

5. *Dulse:*   This can be added raw or slightly toasted to soups, salads, and vegetable, grain and bean dishes at the very end of preparation for extra flavor. It can also be lightly toasted by itself, crumbled and used as a condiment.

6. *Agar-agar:*   This is used as a jelling agent for *kantens* and *aspics*. You can purchase it in the form of bars or powder with the instructions enclosed. (See *Desserts* chapter for *kanten* recipes.)

13. Seasonings, Condiments, Sauces and Dressings ━━━━━━━━━━

Besides your foods and cooking methods, seasonings and condiments play a vital part in the balancing of a meal. As with any other aspect of preparing foods, care must be taken to have enough variety. The chart below is a listing of some of the condiments mentioned in this book. They are categorized into the five tastes and making sure that you use something from each column insures a well rounded meal. Some items fit into more than one category. (Don't over use them, especially the salty items. In most cases, just a light accent is enough.)

SOUR	BITTER	SWEET	PUNGENT	SALTY
Pickles	*Gomashio*	*Miso*	Ginger	*Miso*
Sauerkraut	*Tekka*	*Amazake*	Scallions	*Gomashio*
Umeboshi	Green *nori*	Applesauce	Onions	*Umeboshi*
Shiso leaves	Parsley	Rice syrup	Grated *daikon*	*Shiso* leaves
Rice vinegar	Dandelion	Barley malt	Watercress	*Shio kombu*
Lemon	*Wakame* powder	*Mirin*		*Wakame* powder
	Mustard greens	Raisins		*Tamari* soy sauce
	(pickled)			*Tekka*

Seasonings: ━━

1. *Sea salt:* Salt is one of the building blocks of life and we cannot survive without it. It is one of the basic ingredients of our blood and gives us vitality, strength, and mental clarity. Learning how to adjust salt intake and finding its balance with oil and water is an important part of mastering the art of cooking.

   Only use white unrefined sea salt. In commercial table salt, much of the valuable trace minerals have been removed. Sugar (dextrose), magnesium and sodium carbonate, and potassium iodide has been added in their place. It depletes important minerals from our body as well as contributing to high blood pressure, heart problems, kidney disorders and illness in general. Grey sea salt is also not recommended as it can cause excessive tightness in the body.

   The amount of salt that we can take depends on our individual condition, our age, our activities and environment. Physically active people, adults, persons with a more vegetarian based history, and persons that live in a more wet, humid and cold climate can take more salt. (Babies shouldn't take salt at all. It should be gradually introduced to them as they grow.) Individuals with a history of heavy meat consumption should carefully limit their intake and may even need to abstain for a short period of time. (These are the persons that benefit from vegetarian, raw food, and salt free diets which help to cleanse their bodies. However, after a while, salt and cooked foods should be reintroduced.)

Too much salt can cause hyperactivity, irritability, kidney problems, thirst and anger among other things. Too little can cause poor circulation, mental lethargy, sleepiness, weakness and so on. (Excess salt can also cause these symptoms at times.)

Your meals shouldn't be overwhelmingly salty. Salt should enhance and draw out the natural flavor and sweetness of your foods, not cover them up. Generally, if you're extremely thirsty or crave fatty, rich foods or strong yin such as sugar, ice cream, and so on when you finish your meal, it is an indication that too large a dose of salty (or hot) condiments and dishes may have been consumed. Salt is very yang and attracts much yin, so too much makes it difficult to eat in a centered manner.

Plain salt is not recommended for use at the table. (An exception may be a small pinch of it on your fresh fruits to draw out their sweetness.) It is too strong and difficult to assimilate in that form. Various condiments which substitute for it—such as sea vegetable powders or a mixture of salt and sesame seeds—are recommended. (See the *Condiments* section in this chapter.)

2. *Miso:*   *Miso* is a paste made out of fermented soybeans and sea salt which has been aged for a period of a few months to as long as three years or more. If only a few months old it is light in color and contains less salt. If older, the color becomes a dark brown and more salt is needed to keep it going for that long a time.

    The darker, longer time *miso* is best for healing and is the kind that is assumed when using *miso* is recommended. The best *miso* is at least two summers old. There are three basic kinds now available in natural food stores. (Don't buy *miso* from Oriental food shops. It may be made without using a natural fermenting process and also may contain chemicals and sugars.)

    A. *Hatcho miso:*   This is 100% soybeans and is the darkest, most yang variety. It is especially recommended for the cold winter months.
    B. *Mugi miso:*   This contains barley, is the sweetest of the three and is appropriate all year round as well as being good for medicinal use.
    C. *Genmai (brown rice) or kome (white rice) miso:*   This contains rice. It is lighter and is good for the summer though it can also be

used year round. Use this less often than the first two.

The short term *miso* comes in red, yellow or white. It is sweet, good for the summer and makes delicious sauces and spreads but doesn't have medicinal value.

Buying bulk *miso* is recommended over the packaged variety, especially when one is trying to heal oneself, as it is more alive. When packing, the *miso* has to be pasteurized, otherwise it will keep fermenting and may burst the package.

Keep the *miso* in a cool, dark place and stir it from time to time. (The short term kind should be refrigerated.) If a white color starts to appear on the surface, mix it into the bulk of the *miso*. This substance is a natural bacterial growth and is not harmful. On the contrary, besides adding more minerals and flavor to the *miso*, it is a reassurance that the *miso* is organic and alive.

3. *Tamari soy sauce and/or shoyu:*   This is a liquid by-product of the *miso* making process. It contains fermented soybeans, water, sea salt and sometimes a small amount of wheat. Be very careful to avoid commercial *shoyu* as it is artificially aged and is full of chemicals and coloring. To be on the safe side, purchase soy sauce from natural food stores instead of Oriental ones.

Tamari can be added to just about any kind of dish for extra flavor. There are numerous recipes which use it throughout this book.

Like salt and *miso*, *tamari* should always be cooked into foods, not added afterwards at the table as this can make you very tight and disrupt your digestion. Also, be careful that you don't take too much.

4. *Umeboshi plum, paste and vinegar and shiso leaf pickle:*   *Umeboshi* plums have very strong medicinal value. They purify the bloodstream, detoxify poisons, stimulate appetite, and at times can help to relieve stomachaches, nausea and air sickness. (Take them along whenever you travel.) When someone isn't feeling well, we separate the meat of the plums from the pit, grind it into a paste with a *suribachi* or just chop it very finely and add it to a thick *kuzu* drink (see *Special Needs* chapter) or serve with rice cream.

Umeboshi plums have been pickled in sea salt and *shiso* leaves (to give it that bright red color) for a year or more. They can be added to just about any dish and may be used as a substitute for salt, *tamari* or *miso*. One plum is a delicious condiment with a bowl of rice or other grains. (See *Grains and Grain Products* chapter for a *Rice ball* recipe.)

Recently, *umeboshi* paste and vinegar (leftover juice from making these pickles) have become available. They are very handy to cook with and can be added to your dishes. However, they don't have the strong healing qualities of the plum. Therefore when making *Special Needs* recipes or when trying to relieve a stomachache (for instance) use the whole plum.

Pickled *shiso* leaves are also available by themselves. They can be sliced and added to your dishes in addition to or as a substitute for salt. They are very valuable when dried or baked and ground into a powder for use as a condiment. In this form, they are helpful for neutralizing strong chemicals in your system.

5. *Oil:* Vegetable oils, which are full of polyunsaturated fatty acids, are needed to build new cells and tissues, to keep warm, for vitamins A and E, to maintain proper metabolism and to lubricate skin and hair among other things. However, much of what you need is already found in grains, beans and seeds so the intake of extra oil can be kept to a minimum, especially during the initial few months of healing. A healthy person can have a small amount of extra oil nearly everyday in a side dish of sautéed vegetables or in a sauce or dressing. Even then, one or two tablespoons are adequate to sauté enough vegetables and grains for a whole family. Also, deep-fried foods shouldn't be consumed more than once a week.

Choose unrefined and cold-pressed oils (meaning that the seeds have been pressed below the boiling point and filtered). This has all the vitamins and nutrients intact, is rich in color, retains the flavor and taste of the original seeds, and is somewhat cloudy in appearance. Please avoid refined oils or oils that have been processed at a high temperature.

Animal oils and fats should be totally avoided as they contain high levels of cholesterol which causes hardening of the arteries and heart disease among other things.

To digest more oily foods such as fried rice, accompany them with grated ginger or grated, raw *daikon* or plenty of chopped raw scallions.

Keep your oils in a tightly sealed container in a cool, dark place or in the refrigerator.

Sesame oil, especially the dark variety made from roasted seeds, is the most healthy one to use as it is easiest to digest and more yang than other varieties. Pumpkin seed oil is an occasional variation, also more yang than other oils.

Corn oil (a lighter oil for pastries or pie crusts), safflower, sunflower and olive oil may all be used occasionally once you are in sound health; it is best to avoid them for now.

6. *Brown Rice Vinegar:* This is to be used occasionally. It is delicious in *sushi*, dressings, grain salads and pickles.

7. *Mirin:* This is a cooking wine made from sweet rice. It is delicous in

sweet and sour sauces as well as in beans, vegetables, noodle broths, dressings and marinades. Use this occasionally; it may be avoided initially for several months.

8. *Ginger:* Ginger is a hot, pungent and very delicious root which stimulates the appetite, and activates circulation.

   A small amount of grated ginger spices up your grains, vegetables and noodles. You can extract the juice by squeezing the grated ginger. (The juice is stronger.) Ginger is taken raw or added at the very end of preparations.

9. *Rice syrup and barley malt:* These are the most healthy sweeteners that you can use. They are the honeys of their respective grains and are delicious in desserts or cooked in with *azuki* or black soybeans.

Condiments

Condiments, though we use them very sparingly, are an indispensable part of macrobiotic eating. They add one or more of the following to a meal: color, extra variety and flavor, extra vitamins and minerals, appetite stimulation, balance, zest, and in some cases, medicinal value.

A small amount of various condiments may be used everyday to accompany your grains. They allow individuals to adjust their intake of salt, minerals or oils to fit their own needs. They are easy to overuse so watch out for this, especially when dealing with the more saltier varieties such as *gomashio* or *tekka*.

Gomashio
(The most commonly used condiment in the macrobiotic diet. It is a perfect balance of salt and oil.)

14–16 Tbsps. black or white sesame seeds
1 Tbsp. sea salt

Dry-roast sea salt in a skillet until it becomes shiny. (Roasting releases moisture in the salt and this helps to make a fluffier *gomashio*.) Place it into a *suribachi*, take the pestle and gently grind it until it becomes a fine powder.

Wash and rinse the sesame seeds and drain them in a fine wire mesh strainer. Place them (they should still be wet) in a skillet and dry-roast them until they pop, emit a nutty fragrance and can be crushed very easily between the thumb and index fingers. Be careful that you don't burn them.

Place the seeds into the *suribachi* with the salt and grind them together until the seeds are half crushed and are all coated with salt. Make gentle circular motions using the grooves on the sides of the *suribachi*. When the *gomashio* cools off, place it into an airtight glass or ceramic container. (If it is still warm, moisture will collect inside the container and cause easy spoilage.) Sprinkle this over your grains and vegetables.

Sesame seeds are high in calcium, protein, iron, phosphorous, vitamin A and niacin. For variety, add sea vegetable powder or *shiso* leaf powder instead of salt. (See *Wakame Powder* and *Shiso Leaf Powder* recipes below.)

Shio Kombu

> **8 long strips (about 12″) *kombu***
> **Enough liquid to cover (50% water and 50% *tamari* soy sauce)**

Cut the *kombu* into 1″ squares with scissors and soak them in water/*tamari* soy sauce for 1–2 days. Place them into an uncovered pot, add enough water/*tamari* soy sauce to cover, bring to a boil, immediately turn the flame to low, place a heat deflector underneath and slowly simmer for a couple of hours until most of the liquid has evaporated. Since this is very strong, have only one or two pieces at every meal.

Nori Condiment

> **10 sheets of *nori* broken or cut into small pieces**
> **1 cup spring water**
> **½ Tbsp. *tamari* soy sauce**

Bring all the ingredients to a boil in a small covered pot, turn the flame to low and slowly simmer for about 20–30 minutes or until most of the liquid has boiled away, leaving a paste of *nori*.

Wakame/Rice Vinegar Condiment

> **1 cup *wakame* soaked and sliced**
> **2 Tbsps. brown rice vinegar**
> **2 Tbsps. soaking or fresh water**
> **2 Tbsps. *tamari* soy sauce**

Cook as in the *nori* condiment.

Wakame Powder

Roast some *wakame* in the oven at 350° F. for 10–15 minutes or until it is crisp but not burnt. Grind and crush it into a fine powder in a *suribachi*. Dulse and *kombu* powder can also be made this way. This may be ground with sesame seeds; in this case, use a proportion of 4–8:1.

Shiso Leaf Powder

1 cup of *shiso* leaves chopped very finely. Dry-roast *shiso* in a skillet
or in the oven at 350° F. until it dries out. Then grind it into a
powder. This can be combined with seeds, sea vegetable powder or
both.

Sauces and Dressings:

It is generally best to use sauces and dressings sparingly. Properly prepared, most good macrobiotic dishes are beauful and delicious enough
to stand on their own. However, it is a nice addition at times, particularly
with more bland or lighter dishes and they can add extra dynamics, like
condiments, without covering up the taste and other qualities of the dish
they accompany.

Kuzu Sauce

    1–1½ cups soup or vegetable stock
    1 Tbsp. *kuzu* dissolved in a small amount of water
    ***Tamari* soy sauce to taste**
    ***Optional:* 2–3 pinches grated ginger**

Bring dissolved *kuzu* and soup stock to a boil, lower the flame,
simmer and stir until the *kuzu* becomes transparent. Add the *tamari*
and ginger and place this over grains or vegetables.

Fig. 35   *Kuzu*

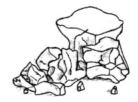

Kuzu Sauce with Vegetables

    ½ carrot cut into thin matchsticks
    1 onion thinly sliced
    2 cups water or soup stock
    2–2½ Tbsps. *kuzu* dissolved in a small amount of water

    ***Tamari* soy sauce to taste**
    ***Optional:* A couple pinches of grated ginger**

Bring vegetables and soup stock to a boil, turn the flame down and
simmer until the vegetables are soft. Add the diluted *kuzu* and stir
until it becomes transparent. Add the *tamari* and optional ginger.

Garnishes

To garnish your dishes you can use *nori*, scallions, parsley, raw onions, sautéed vegetables, red radishes, boiled greens, lemons, grated vegetables, croutons, sliced fruits, roasted seeds and nuts and so on.

Umeboshi Dressing

>2 tsps. *umeboshi* paste
>½ cup or a little more water
>½ tsp. diced onions

Grind paste, onions and water in a *suribachi* into a purée. You can use this for boiled salads, boiled *tofu* or other milder dishes.

Tofu Dressing

>1 cube *tofu*
>1 tsp. *umeboshi* paste
>1 Tbsp. grated onion
>2 tsps. more of water

Purée all the ingredients in a *suribachi*.

Miso Dressing

>3 Tbsps. puréed *miso*
>1 Tbsp. grated onion
>2 Tbsps. brown rice vinegar
>6 Tbsps. water
>Some chopped scallions

Purée all the ingredients together except the scallion which you mix in last.

Tamari/Ginger/Vinegar Dressing

>2 Tbsps. *tamari* soy sauce
>½–1 cup water
>¼ tsp. grated ginger
>8 Tbsps. brown rice vinegar

Mix all the ingredients together.

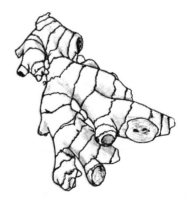

Fig. 36   Ginger

For variations:

1) *Miso* and *tamari* are interchangeable.
2) *Umeboshi* is interchangeable with *miso* and *tamari* though it doesn't go well with rice vinegar or lemon.
3) Ginger, onions, parsley, scallions and chives are interchangeable and can be used singularly or in combination. Using more than two at one time can get a bit too complicated.
4) Lemon can be substituted for rice vinegar.
5) Heated sesame oil may be left out or added.

14. Desserts ━━━━━━━━━━━━━━━━━━━━━━━━━

You can make delicious desserts using squash, sweet grains or *azuki* beans as a base, rather than fruit or flour. The best sweeteners for your health are:

1. *Amazake*, a drink or a pudding made out of fermented sweet rice and a starter called *koji*, also made out of rice. It can be consumed as it is as well as being added to other dessert recipes.
2. Rice syrup.
3. Barley malt syrup.
4. Chestnuts.
5. *Mirin*, a cooking wine made from sweet rice. It is used more in regular cooking than in desserts.
6. Raisins and other dried fruits such as apples, peaches, pears, apricots, currants, and cherries.
7. Fresh seasonal fruits cooked.
8. Apple juice and cider.

Agar-agar and *kuzu* are natural thickeners you can use in place of eggs, gelatin, and the like.

For more extensive recipes on cookies, cakes, muffins and so on, refer to other macrobiotic cookbooks. Since this book deals mainly with the healing process, I didn't include these less healthful types of desserts.

Amazake

(Also sold ready-made in some natural food stores.)

4 cups sweet brown rice
$\frac{1}{2}$ cup *koji* (sold in some natural food stores)
8 cups water

Soak the rice overnight and pressure-cook for 30 minutes. When done, place it into a glass bowl and as soon as it becomes cool enough to handle, mix in the *koji*, cover with a towel and put it in a warm place. An oven with just the pilot light on or the radiator will do. Let this ferment for 4–8 hours. Mix it once in a while to help dissolve the *koji*. The fermentation is done when bubbles start to appear on the surface together with a sweet taste. It becomes sweeter and sweeter up to a certain point and then it starts to turn sour. Catch it when it's sweet, place it back into a pot, bring it to a boil, add a pinch of sea salt and turn it off as soon as it starts to bubble.

You can use it as it is or you can blend it in a food mill. For a delicious drink, after you blend it, add a small amount of water and optional grated ginger, bring to a boil and serve. Or you can let it cool off to make a refreshing cold beverage.

To keep the *amazake* for a longer time, simmer it over a low flame with a heat deflector underneath until it becomes a little bit brown.

Basic *Amazake* Pudding

4 cups *amazake* drink
6 Tbsps. *kuzu,* dissolved in a small amount of water
2 pinches sea salt
Optional: 1/4 cup raisins

Place all ingredients into a pot, and bring to a boil while stirring constantly with a wooden spoon to avoid lumping and burning. Then simmer for about 3 minutes, pour into a serving plate, let it set, garnish and serve. If it jelled properly, you can slice it into several squares. Serves 8.

Chestnut Sweet Rice

2 cups sweet rice
1/2 cup dried chestnuts
3 cups spring water
2 pinches sea salt

Wash the chestnuts (sort out discolored ones) and dry-roast them for about 5 minutes in a skillet over a medium low flame. Stir with a wooden spoon, making sure that they don't burn. Put them in a pressure-cooker with the sweet rice and cook as in the *Basic Brown Rice* recipe. Serves 4–6.

Sweet *Azuki* Beans

1 cup *azuki* beans
1 cup chestnuts
1/8 cup raisins (or 1/2 cup *ame* rice syrup
5 cups water
1/2 tsp. sea salt

Soak the *azuki* and chestnut for 6–8 hours or overnight. Place all the ingredients except salt into a pressure-cooker and pressure-cook for 40–45 minutes. Let the pressure come down completely, uncover, add salt, bring to a boil again, turn flame to low, and simmer for another 5–10 minutes. Or you can simmer for a longer time, until all the excess liquid has boiled away. (That would make this really sweet.) Serves 4–6.

Ohagi

- 2 cups sweet rice
- 2 cups chestnuts
- 7 cups spring water
- 4 pinches sea salt
- ½ cup black sesame seeds
- 1 Tbsp. *tamari* soy sauce

Dry-roast the chestnuts and pressure-cook them in 5 cups of water and 2 pinches of sea salt for 45–50 minutes. When done, blend it into a purée with a food mill.

Wash and dry-roast the black sesame seeds until they start to pop and emit a nutty fragrance. Put them into a bowl and pour the *tamari* on them.

Meanwhile, pressure-cook the sweet rice in 3 cups of water and 2 pinches of sea salt for 40–45 minutes. When it's done, vigorously pound the rice with a wooden pestle until the grains are half broken (in 15–20 minutes). Wet your hands and form the rice into small balls.

Coat some of the balls in sesame seeds and *tamari* by rolling them in the seeds. Coat the other ones in the chestnut purée by molding the purée onto them. Place them onto serving plates, creating some kind of attractive decoration with the two different kinds of balls and some garnish. Serves 4.

You can also coat them with either the *Sweet Azuki Beans* dish mentioned above, some dry-roasted, finely chopped walnuts mixed with *tamari* or a squash purée.

Couscous Cake with Pumpkin Seeds and Raisins

- 2 cups couscous
- 1 cup raisins
- ½ cup dry-roasted pumpkin seeds
- ¾ cup water or apple juice
- 1 pinch sea salt

Steam couscous for 5–7 minutes, remove, fluff it up with a fork and add pumpkin seeds to it.

Boil and simmer raisins, water or juice, and salt for 3 minutes. Remove and mix all the ingredients together and press them into a cake pan. Let cool, slice and serve. Serves 6.

Sweet *Kuzu*

(See *Special Needs* Chapter)

Dried Apricot *Kanten*

    2 cups dried apricots, soaked a couple of hours
    4 cups apple juice (or 2 cups juice & 2 cups water)
    ⅛ tsp. sea salt
    1 bar agar-agar or 6 Tbsps. agar-agar flakes
    1 Tbsp. *kuzu*, diluted in a little water

Bring apricots, juice (or water and juice) and sea salt to a boil,
turn the flame to low and simmer until the apricots become soft.
Add the diluted *kuzu* and the agar-agar and stir until the *kuzu*
becomes clear and the agar dissolves. Place a little coating of
water into a mold (so that the *kanten* will be easy to remove later
on) and place everything into it and let it sit until it sets. Vary
with other fruits. Fresh fruits should be added at or towards the
end of simmering. Nuts can also be added. Serves 8.

Applesauce

    8 apples, cored, peeled and sliced
    Water to keep them from burning, about ½ "–1" deep
    2 Tbsps. rice syrup (*optional*)
    2 pinches sea salt
    1 Tbsp. *kuzu* (optional: for a very yin condition)

Bring everything to a boil, then turn the flame down and simmer
until the apples become soft. Purée in a food mill and serve. Serves
2–3.

Pie Crust (Regular)

    4 cups whole wheat pastry flour
    1 cup corn oil
    Just enough cold water to hold it together
    1 tsp. sea salt

Mix flour and salt, add the oil while stirring with a fork until little
balls and lumps start to form. Gradually add water until you can
form a ball of dough as you keep stirring with the fork. This dough
should not be sticky and watery. If it is, sprinkle in some more flour.
   Separate the dough in two. Take a rolling pin and one of the
halves of dough and roll it out flat in between two sheets of wax
paper. You can work on top of a cutting board. If the bottom paper
slides around too much, wet it's underside slightly. You can also
sprinkle some flour or brush a little oil where the paper and dough
make contact to prevent them from sticking together. However, if
the dough isn't so wet to begin with, this shouldn't be much of a
problem. Carefully peel off the paper on top, turn the dough upside

down and center it into a pie plate. Then peel off the other side. If you are making an open face pie, first trim away the excess dough that hangs over the edge with a knife. Then with your fork, poke some air holes in the crust to let steam escape (otherwise it will get bubbly) and fasten the outer rim of the crust onto the pie plate by indenting little grooves all around the edge. Use the other half of the dough for another pie. Bake the empty shell for 10 minutes at 375° F. Then take it out, add the filling and bake again until the crust turns a golden brown.

If you are making a pie with a top crust, after inserting the bottom one, add the filling, roll out the other half of the dough and place it on top in the same manner as you did before. Trim away the excess dough. Again, with the fork, poke some air holes in the top crust and seal the upper and lower crusts together by indenting grooves around the outer rim. Then bake.

You can roll out the leftover dough, slice it and bake the pieces as cookies.

Pie Crust (*Mochi*)
(This is a much healthier alternative to regular pie crust but is only practical for open faced pies.)

Cook and pound some sweet rice as in the *Mochi* recipe but then, instead of making the *mochi*, oil a pie plate and press the rice into it and shape a pie crust. Then bake as usual. This doesn't need to be prebaked before adding your filling.

Apple Pie

   10–12 apples, cored, sliced and peeled
   ¼ cup *ame* syrup or barley malt
   2 Tbsps. arrowroot flour
   ¼ cup water
   2–3 pinches sea salt

Boil and simmer all the ingredients together until the apples become soft, stirring often to prevent burning and lumping. Cool it off, place in a pie shell and bake. For variations, use other dried or fresh fruit, sweet vegetables such as squash and/or chestnuts.

Fish should be eaten as fresh as possible, preferably the same day it is caught or at least the same day it is purchased. Choose more slow moving, soft white-meat and yin fish such as sole, flounder, haddock, carp and so on, as opposed to more active, red-meat varieties such as tuna, salmon, swordfish, and the like. Temporarily avoid shellfish such as clams, oysters, mussels, shrimp, lobsters and crabs.

It is best for skin allergic persons to avoid all fish entirely, at least for several months or until symptoms have improved.

Eat two or three times the regular amount of hard leafy greens when including fish in a meal to help balance, it's strong yang energies. Grated *daikon* with a few drops of *tamari* soy sauce and a bit of grated ginger will help neutralize any possible toxic side-effects of the fish. A few drops of lemon is helpful and a slice of lemon is a beautiful garnish as well.

Clear Fish Soup

> **1–2 fillets of sole (or other white-meat fish)**
> **1 cup *wakame* soaked & cut into 1″ slices**
> **1 bunch watercress, previously boiled for 1 second**
> **3 *shiitake* mushrooms, soaked and sliced**
> **5–6 cups *kombu* stock (add *shiitake* soaking water)**
> ***Tamari* soy sauce to taste**

Bring *wakame*, *shiitake* and *kombu* stock to a boil, turn the flame down and simmer for a few minutes until the *wakame* and *shiitake* soften. Cut the fish into 1½″–2″ pieces and add them to the soup with *tamari* to taste and simmer for 1–2 minutes or until the fish turns white. Ladle the soup into individual serving bowls and garnish with the watercress. Serves 6–8.

Fish Stew

> **1 lb. cod (or other white-meat fish)**
> **12 thin slices lotus root**
> **9 ½″ *daikon* rounds, cut in half**
> **2 12″ strips *kombu*, soaked and softened**
> **6 cups water (including *kombu* soaking water)**
> **4–5 tsps. *kuzu*, dissolved in a little bit of water**
> ***Tamari* soy sauce to taste**
> **3 chopped scallions**

Cut the *kombu* into 1″ squares and boil in the soaking water until soft. Add the vegetables and the rest of the water and boil and simmer until they are soft. Cut the fish in 2″ slices and add to the soup with the *tamari* and *kuzu*. Stir and simmer 3–5 minutes until the soup thickens a bit. Garnish with chopped scallions and serve. Serves 6–8.

Koi Koku (Carp Soup)

(This very strong soup increases strength and vitality. In Japan it is served to mothers who have just given birth. It is delicious in the winter and medicinal for those who have become very weak.)

> 1 small carp (about 2 lbs.)
> Equal volume of thinly shaved burdock
> ½–1 cup *bancha* tea twigs and leaves (already used to make tea)
> Enough liquid to cover, ⅓ *bancha* & ⅔ water
> Grated ginger
> *Miso* to taste, puréed
> Clean, 100% cotton cheesecloth

Buy a fresh carp, preferably a live one and ask the fish seller to kill it for you. Also ask him to carefully (so as not to break it) remove the gallbladder and the yellow bitter thyroid bone. Leave the rest of the fish intact.

At home, chop the whole fish (bones, head, fins and all) into 1″ slices.

Make a sack out of the cheesecloth and put the used *bancha* twigs inside like a tea bag. This helps to soften the fish bones.

Place all the ingredients (including the sack of used tea twigs) except the *miso* into a pressure cooker. Pressure-cook for 1 hour. Bring down the pressure, take off the lid, add the ginger and *miso* to taste, simmer for 5 minutes and serve. Garnish with chopped scallions. Serves 6–8.

Steamed Trout

> 1 trout, cleaned
> 3 *shiitake* mushrooms, soaked & left whole
> 4–5 broccoli flowerettes
> 6″ piece *kombu*, soaked
> Lemon slices
> Grated *daikon*

Make shallow diagonal slits on both sides of the fish. Place *kombu* on the bottom of a ceramic cooking bowl and place the fish and *shiitake* on top. Place the lid on top.

In a large pot, bring a ½″ layer of water to a boil, then place the ceramic bowl containing the fish into the pot. Steam for 12 minutes, add the broccoli, steam for 3 more minutes, remove from the pot and serve with lemon slices and grated *daikon*. Serves 3–4.

Baked Flounder

    1 flounder, washed
    3 Tbsps. white *miso*
    2 Tbsps. *mirin*
    3 Tbsps. *kombu* stock
    Grated *daikon*

Place the flounder on an oiled baking dish. Make several shallow diagonal slits along the top of it and bake 7–10 minutes.

Meanwhile, puree and mix the *miso*, *kombu* stock and *mirin* in a *suribachi*. Pour this over the baking fish when it is 70 percent done, bake another 5 minutes and serve with grated *daikon*. Serves 1–2.

16. Beverages ━━━━━━━━━━━━━━━━━

It is best to drink only when we are thirsty. Most of us drink out of habit, whether we want to or not (as we do with food). If you are always thirsty some of the dietary reasons may include:

1) **Overconsumption of salt.**
2) **Overconsumption of animal products.**
3) **Overconsumption of dry, baked and or floury foods.**
4) **Overconsumption of spices**
5) **Overconsumtion of food in general.**
6) **Not chewing enough**
7) **Lack of fresh, light dishes**
8) **Excess of sea vegetables**

Good quality water, such as spring or well water is the best to use. Avoid distilled or highly chemicalized tap water as much as possible.

It is also best to avoid iced or cold drinks (even water) as they can shock and paralyze your digestive system and harden fat accumulations in the body.

The beverages used on a daily basis don't contain caffeine, sugar, carbonation, artificial color, preservatives, stimulants or alcohol (particularly the hard liquor varieties). If you are following a more general Standard Diet you can bend this a bit and have small occasional quantities of more yin, good quality drinks such as green tea, beer, *saké* and mint teas. But on a diabetes or hypoglycemic healing diet, these items are best avoided.

The recipes in the *Special Needs* chapter are to be used only when really necessary and for a short period of time.

Bancha Twig Tea (*Kukicha*)
(For daily use, the brown rice of beverages.)

1–2 Tbsps. *bancha* twigs
1½ quarts water

Twig tea generally comes pre-roasted. If it isn't, dry-roast the whole package of twigs and leaves in a skillet for 3–4 minutes while stirring gently with a wooden spoon. Take out the 1–2 tablespoons that you are going to use and store the rest, after cooling, in an airtight jar until needed.

Add twigs to cold water, bring them to a boil, reduce the flame to low and simmer 10–15 minutes, depending on how light or dark you want it. While serving the tea into individual cups, use a bamboo tea strainer (available in natural or Oriental food stores) to strain out the twigs. A regular metal strainer can be used as an alternative. The twigs may be reused several times until they lose their strength but make it fresh on a regular basis.

Kukicha contains no caffeine, artificial colorings or dyes and is not aromatic. It aids digestion and helps to settle an acidic stomach as it is alkaline in nature. (Most teas are acidic.)

Kukicha or *bancha* is made from the twigs and leaves of an older, matured tea bush, named *ban* in Japanese. (*Cha* is the Japanese word for tea. Hence, saying "*bancha* tea" is really calling it *ban* tea tea.)

The same bush also supplies some green tea which is made from the topmost and youngest, greenest leaves. This tea is delicious but contains much caffeine and is not recommended for regular use. As the bush becomes older, the caffeine content begins to decrease and finally disappears. Harvesting different sections of the plant and at different stages in it's growth produces a variety of teas.

Homemade Grain Teas
(Good for daily or regular use.)

To make grain teas, wash and dry-roast one of the following; rice, millet, oats, barley, wheat, etc., in a dry skillet. Use a wooden spoon to stir. Store what you don't need in an airtight container, after cooling, for later use. Take 2 Tbsps. for 1½–2 quarts of water and boil and simmer as in *bancha* tea.

Mugicha (Roasted Unhulled Barley Tea)
(Good for daily or regular use.)

2 Tbsps. *mugicha* (available in natural food stores)
1½–2 quarts water

Place the *mugicha* in cold water, bring it to a boil, reduce the flame to low and simmer several minutes, the time depending on how strong you want it.

Yannoh/Grain Coffee/Root Coffee
(For more "occasional use")

4 tsp. *yannoh*
4 cups water

Bring *yannoh* and 4 cups of cold water to a boil. Immediately reduce the flame (as it will boil over), and simmer for several minutes.

Yannoh is sold in natural food stores but may be difficult to find. (When buying grain coffee, make sure that it doesn't contain fruits or more yin vegetables such as beets.) You can make your own homemade *yannoh* by washing, separately dry-roasting (till a nutty fragrance is emitted) and grinding.

Yannoh

3 cups brown rice
2½ cups wheat
1½ cups *azuki* beans
2 cups chickpeas
1 cup chicory root

When it's cool, store it in an airtight glass jar. You can experiment and vary different proportions of grains, beans and vegetables (like burdock or dandelion root) with chicory to find a winning combination. One hundred percent dandelion root coffee can be delicious.

Azuki Bean Tea
(For occasionally use, often used medicinally.)

1 cup *azuki* beans
3–4 cups water
1 piece *kombu*

Put *kombu* in the bottom of a pan, then add *azuki* beans and water. Boil, reduce the flame to low and simmer until the water becomes a rich red. This is good for tight kidneys. Have one cup a day for 3 days to help loosen them.

Kombu Tea
(For "occasional use.")

1 strip *kombu*, 6″
2 cups water

Boil the *kombu* and water until only 1 cup of liquid remains.

Mu Tea
(For "occasional use" only.)

1 tea bag of *Mu* tea (sold in natural food stores)
4 cups water

Boil, reduce flame and simmer for 10 minutes. *Mu* tea is made of 9–16 different herbs. The mixture was concocted by my teacher, George Oshawa, the man who first introduced macrobiotic principles to the Western countries.

Umeboshi **Tea**
(For "occasional use.")

> **3–4 *umeboshi* plums**
> **1½–2 quarts water**
> ***Optional:* 1 or 2 *shiso* leaves**

Separate the meat of the *umeboshi* from the pits and tear them into several pieces. Add the *umeboshi* meat and pits to the water and bring everything to a boil. Turn the flame to low and simmer for 20–30 minutes. This is delicious when cooled in the summer. It also helps to reduce thirst and replaces minerals lost by excessive sweating.

Leftover Vegetable Juice
("Occasional use")

You can drink the leftover water from boiling or pressure-cooking vegetables. Just make sure that there isn't a lot of concentrated salt in the water.

Vegetable and Fruit Juices

The juice of any "regular use" vegetable or seasonal fruit on the *Standard Macrobiotic Die* list may be taken occasionally. In the winter it is preferable to heat juices up, especially the yinner fruit juices. It is better for allergic persons to avoid this for a few months until their condition clears up.

17. Special Needs ━━━━━━━━━━━━━━

You can supplement your meals with some home remedies. For more information about their use, read the companion book (*Macrobiotic Health Education Series*) as well as the chapter on *Dietary Adjustments for Diabetes and Hypoglycemia* in this book.

Internal remedies: ━━━━━━━━━━━━━━━━━━━━━

Agar-agar with *Ame* or Barley Malt
(To relieve constipation.)

> 1½ Tbsp. agar-agar flakes
> 1 Tbsp. *ame* rice syrup or barley malt
> 1 cup spring water
> 1 pinch sea salt

Bring all the ingredients to a boil, then turn the flame down and simmer 5–10 minutes. Take it off the stove, cool it and let it jell before you take it.

Ame-kuzu Drink
(For coughing attacks and asthmatic breathing problems.)

> 1 tsp. *kuzu*
> 1 Tbsp. *ame* rice syrup or barley malt
> 1 cup spring water

Dissolve the *kuzu* in 2 teaspoons of water until it becomes a liquid and put it into a pot with 1 cup of water and either *ame* rice syrup or barley malt. Stirring constantly with a wooden spoon, bring this to a boil, turn the flame to low, simmer 10–15 minutes and serve hot.

Amazake Drink
(For coughing attacks and breathing problems.)

Boil 1–2 cups of *amazake* drink and drink hot.

Bancha Tea with *Ame* Syrup
(For coughing attacks and breathing problems.)

Boil a cup of *bancha* tea with 1 tablespoon of *ame* rice syrup or barley malt and drink hot.

Grated Lotus Juice

(Relieves coughing and dissolves excess mucus. Especially helpful for asthma or allergic bronchitis and hay fever.)

> ½ cup fresh lotus root, grated
> Equal amount of water
> 1 pinch sea salt or a couple drops of *tamari* soy sauce
> 1 pinch ginger, freshly grated
> Cheesecloth (6″ by 6″)

Form a sack with the cheesecloth, place the grated lotus root inside and squeeze out as much liquid as you can into a small pot. Add water and salt or *tamari*, bring this to a boil, turn the flame to low, simmer for 5–8 minutes, add the ginger and drink hot.

Lotus Root Powder Tea

(Sold in natural food stores. Used when fresh lotus [see above] can't be found. It works but is not as effective.)

> 1 tsp. lotus root powder
> ½ cup water
> 1 pinch sea salt
> 1 pinch ginger, grated

Bring lotus powder, salt and water to a boil over a low flame. Then simmer for a few seconds, add the ginger and drink hot.

Ume-Sho-Kuzu

(Strengthens digestion, energizes.)

> 1 heaping tsp. *kuzu*
> 1 tsp. *tamari* soy sauce
> 1 *umeboshi* plum
> ⅛ tsp. ginger, freshly grated
> 1 cup spring water

Grate the ginger and chop the meat of the *umeboshi* plum and put them aside. Dissolve the *kuzu* in 2 teaspoons of water until it becomes a liquid and add it to a small pot with 1 cup of water. Bring this to a boil and then turn the flame to low as you keep stirring constantly with a wooden spoon. When the milky white color turns transparent, add the *tamari*, *umeboshi* and ginger. Drink this immediately while it's hot.

Lotus Seeds and *Kombu*

> ½ cup lotus seeds, soaked overnight
> 3″ strip *kombu*, soaked & cut into thin matchsticks
> A few drops of *tamari* soy sauce
> Enough water to cover the seeds

Bring the lotus seeds, *kombu* and water to a boil, then turn the flame to low and simmer for about 30 minutes or until the seeds and *kombu* become soft. Then add a few drops of *tamari* to taste and simmer another 5 minutes. You can also use fresh or dried lotus root.

External treatments:

Ginger Compress
(Helps circulation, dissolves mucus, cysts, tumors, etc.)

> **6 Tbsps. grated ginger**
> **1 gallon water**
> **Cheesecloth 6″ by 6″**
> **Rubber gloves**
> **3 cotton towels**
> ***Optional:* hot plate**
> **(A person to give the treatment. It's awkward and not relaxing to do it yourself.)**

Bring a pot of water to a boil and turn the flame off. Meanwhile, make a sack out of cheesecloth, place the grated ginger inside, and tie the open end into a knot to close it. Immediately after turning off the flame and the bubbles have disappeared, squeeze as much ginger liquid as you can out of the sack and into the pan. Then, place the whole bag inside. The point is to put the ginger in as hot a water as possible without boiling it, as that would cancel its effectiveness.

Lay the patient down on a bed or some cushions and let him/her relax. Put on some rubber gloves. Holding both ends of a cotton towel, dip as much of the towel as you can into the water. Wring it out and place it on the affected area of the patient's body. If it's too hot, shake it a bit before placing it on. Ideally it should be as hot as one can stand. Cover this with a dry cotton towel to keep it warm for a longer time. Place another towel in the water and when the first towel has cooled off, wring this one and exchange it with the first. Again, cover with the dry towel. Continue alternating the towels until the area being treated becomes red. You can reheat (but not boil) the water a bit if it becomes too cool.

This treatment, which softens stagnated tumors, mucus deposits, and the like, is sometimes followed by some kind of plaster which helps to draw out the poisons that have been loosened.

Buckwheat Plaster

(Draws out excess fluid from swollen areas.)

> **Buckwheat flour**
> **Enough hot water to form a hard, stiff dough**
> **5–10% grated ginger**
> **Clean cotton linen**

Precede the plaster with a 5 minute application of ginger compress on the swollen area. Form a dough with the flour, hot water and ginger, and place a ½″ layer on the affected area. Cover and tie it on with a strip of linen. Replace the buckwheat every 4 hours. The swelling should go down after several applications or at the most after 2–3 days.

Lotus Root Plaster

(Draws out excess mucus, especially from the sinuses, lungs and bronchi.)

> **75–85% grated fresh lotus root**
> **10–15% pastry flour**
> **5–10% grated ginger**
> **Cotton linen**

Mix these ingredients and spread them ½″ thick onto a linen cloth. Apply the plaster directly to the skin on the area you are treating. Tie and keep this on for a few hours or overnight and repeat this for a few days. It's helpful to do a ginger compress beforehand.

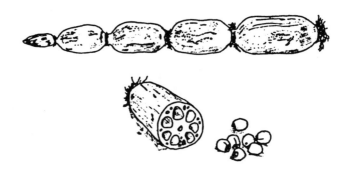

Fig. 37   Lotus root and seeds

Mustard Plaster

(Stimulates circulation and loosens stagnation.)

> Mustard powder
> Enough hot water to make a paste
> Paper towels
> Two thick cotton towels

Make a paste with the powder and hot water and spread it onto a paper towel. Sandwich this in between two thick towels and place on the affected area. (*Don't Put the Mustard Directly onto the Skin.*) Remove this when the skin becomes red and hot. Wipe the skin clean.

Daikon Leaves Hip Bath

(For female sexual organ troubles.)

> 4–5 bunches dried *daikon* leaves
> 4–5 quarts water
> 1 handful sea salt
> A bathtub of waist level hot water
> A towel

Dry several bunches of fresh *daikon* tops or greens in the shade until they become dry and brittle. (Use turnip greens if *daikon* isn't available.)

Boil the dried tops with the handful of salt until the 4–5 quarts of water turns brown. Straining out the leaves, pour the liquid into the bathtub. The water in the tub (make it hot) should come up to waist level. With a towel covering the upper part of your body, sit in the tub until the whole body becomes warm and begins to sweat (about 10 minutes). Do this for as many days as needed. Follow the bath with a *bancha* tea douche (see below).

Bancha Tea Douche

(For female sex organs.)

> Enough luke-warm *bancha* tea for douching
> ½ tsp. sea salt
> Juice from half a lemon or equivalent amount of brown rice vinegar

Combine all the ingredients and use as a douche after taking the *daikon* leaves hip bath.

Greens with Bran Plaster

(Helps to reduce discomfort from skin irritation or inflammation.)

50% rice bran
50% finely chopped, raw, green leafy vegetables
A little water to help make a paste
Cotton linen

Crush the hard leafy, chopped greens (such as collards, kale, watercress, etc.) in a *suribachi* until they turn into a pulp. Combine with the bran and some water to make a paste. Apply on the feverish area and remove it when the paste becomes warm or hot.

Greens with *Nori* Plaster

(Also helps to reduce discomfort from skin irritation or inflammation.)

Finely chopped, raw, green leafy vegetables.
A few sheets of *nori*

Crush the greens (such as collards, kale, watercress, etc.) and *nori* in a *suribachi* until they become a pulp and apply this on the feverish area until the paste becomes warm or hot.

Tofu Plaster

1 cake fresh *tofu*
Equivalent amount of finely diced cabbage
Enough whole wheat flour to hold it together, about 10–20% of the plaster
1 tsp. grated ginger

Grind the *tofu* and cabbage into a paste in a *suribachi*. Add the ginger and flour and place this plaster mixture onto a cheesecloth or cotton cloth, forming a sack with the *tofu* inside. Put this onto the forehead or any other affected area using the cheesecloth to tie it in place. When the mixture becomes warm, perhaps every 2–3 hours, exchange it for a fresh application.

Rice Bran Wash

Take two handfuls of bran. Make a sack for it out of a cotton cloth or cheesecloth (several layers thick), put in the bran and tie it tightly. Use this to scrub your body when you take a bath or shower. It can be used several times until it starts to spoil. This is also good for skin rashes.

Glossary

Agar-agar—A white gelatin made from sea vegetable, used for making *kanten*. You can get it in bars or flakes.

Ame—A natural grain honey derived from rice, barley or wheat.

Amazake—A sweet porridge or drink made from fermented sweet rice. You can make this at home or get it in some natural food stores.

Arame—A variety of sea vegetable.

Arepas—Corn cake made from *masa* corn dough.

Arrowroot—A finely ground white flour, used as a thickener, similar to *kuzu* and corn starch.

Azuki beans—Small, red beans. They're good for the kidneys.

Bancha—Tea made from a tea bush which is at least three years old. It helps digestion, and is good for daily use.

Burdock—A long, thin, dark, black root which grows all over the states as well as in other parts of the world. It gives one strength and stamina.

Couscous—A partially refined cracked wheat. It's light and cooks quickly. It is good for summer cooking.

Daikon—A long, thick, white root from the radish family. It is pungent when raw and is sweet when cooked. It is an excellent cleanser and purifier of blood by cutting down on excess fat deposits. Grated raw and with a drop of *tamari* soy sauce, it is a good garnish with oily, greasy foods, making them more digestible.

Dulse—A variety of sea vegetable harvested in Maine, among other places.

Fu—Derived from wheat gluten, you can buy it in natural food stores in either flat, thin sheets or in round donut shapes. When dry it is like a cracker but when cooked it is more like a noodle. A fun food.

Ginger—A hot, pungent, gnarly-looking, flesh colored root. It adds zest to your dishes and also helps circulation whether taken internally or applied externally as in a ginger compress.

Ginger compress—An external treatment made from grated ginger and hot water. It stimulates ciruclation and unblocks stagnation (see *recipe*).

Gomashio—A condiment made from roasted sesame seeds and sea salt.

Hijiki—A black stringy variety of sea vegetable.

Hokkaido squash—A delicous squash, similar to buttercup.

Jinenjo—A very hardy, long, flesh colored, mountain root potato. When grated it becomes a sticky mass and can be eaten with grains or you can slice it and add it to vegetable dishes. It gives one strength.

Kanten—A jello type food made from agar-agar. It makes a great light dessert when made with fruit and fruit juice. It's also used for aspics.

Kasha—Buckwheat groats.

Kinpira—Thinly sliced or shaved, sautéed burdock dish with or without carrots and seasoned with *tamari* soy sauce.

Koji—Rice which has been innoculated with a form of bacteria. It is used as a starter for making *amazake, saké, miso* and *tamari* soy sauce.

Kombu—A long, smooth, flat, thick variety of sea vegetable used in soup stocks, vegetable, beans, grain dishes and condiments.

Kukicha—Another name for *bancha*.

Kuzu—A starch made from the root of the *kuzu* plant (called *kudzu* in the States) which is used as a thickener in vegetables dishes as well as for medicinal purposes. When you buy it, it looks like little white rocks.

Lotus root—A tubular, flesh colored root from the water lily family. It is hollowed out by several lengthwise airholes. It's good for the respiratory system and helps to unclog the sinuses.

Lotus seeds—Seeds of the above. They look like chickpeas.

Masa—A whole corn dough used as a base for *arepas, tortillas,* porridges and so on. You make it at home but some natural food stores have started carrying already made.

Mirin—A sweet wine made from rice and used in cooking.

Miso—A salty paste made from fermented soybeans with or without grains. Many varieties are available (see *Soup* section).

Mochi—Cakes made from pounded sweet rice which are dried and later used in a variety of dishes. It can be made at home or purchased in a natural food store. Make sure to get the brown rice variety instead of the white.

Mugicha—Tea made from roasted barley.

Natto—Stringy, fermented soybeans which when mixed with scallions, *tamari* soy sauce, grated ginger and *daikon*, makes an excellent companion to a bowl of rice. The taste for it has to be acquired for some people. A good source of protein. It can be homemade or store bought.

Nishime—A method of cooking vegetables with a minimal amount of water.

Nori—A variety of sea vegetable which comes compressed into thin paper-like sheets. It can be used as a garnish, a cover for *sushi* and rice balls and also as a condiment.

Norimaki—A type of *sushi* which is made by rolling *nori*, rice and vegetables together into a long roll with a *sushi* mat.

Ohagi—Little balls of cooked, sweet rice which can be covered with seeds, nuts, or *azuki* beans among other things.

Ojiya—A porridge of soft rice, vegetables and *miso* (sea salt or *tamari* soy sauce can substitute for the *miso*).

Sea salt—Salt from the sea, much healthier than commercial land salt which contains iodine, sugar and chemicals.

Seitan—Wheat gluten which has been boiled (and optionally deep-fried as well) with *tamari* soy sauce, *kombu* and water. It's a good replacement for meat.

Shiitake—A variety of dried mushroom which is helpful in breaking down animal fats within the body. It is used as a soup stock or in vegetable dishes.

Shio kombu—A condiment made from *kombu* and *tamari* soy sauce.

Shiso—Beefsteak plant leaves which are pickled with *umeboshi* plums for added color. It strengthens blood quality and can be used as a condiment.

Soba—Japanese buckwheat noodles.

Somen—An extremely thin variety of Japanese wheat noodles.

Suribachi—A ceramic bowl with grooves and a pestle for grinding and puréeing.

Sushi—Rice formed into little balls and topped with fish or vegetables as well as rolls (*norimaki*) made from *nori*, rice and vegetables.

Sushi mat—Bamboo mat used for making *norimaki sushi*.

Takuan—*Daikon* rice-bran pickles.

Tamari—A name given to naturally made soy sauce to differentiate it from the commercially made, chemicalized ones.

Tekka—A strong condiment made out of burdock, carrots, lotus root, ginger, *miso* and sesame. Available in natural food stores.

Tempeh—Cakes of fermented soybeans, used widely in Indonesia and available in natural food stores. A good source of protein.

Tofu—A white cake made from soybeans and water, also known as bean curd, available fresh or dried.

Udon—Japanese wheat noodles.

Umeboshi—Salty pickled plums. Helps cleanse the blood and aids digestion.

Wakame—A thin, leafy variety of sea vegetable.

Yannoh—Grain beverage sometimes used as a coffee substitute—made from five different grains.

Bibliography

Macrobiotic Health Education Series, Japan Publications.
   a) Kushi, Michio with John D. Mann, *Diabetes and Hypoglycemia*, Tokyo, Japan Publications, 1985
   b) Kushi, Michio with Mark Mead and John D. Mann, *Allergies*, Tokyo, Japan Publications, 1985
Macrobiotic Food and Cooking Series, Japan Publications
Kushi, Aveline with Rosalind Rhodes, *Cooking for Health. Allergies*, Tokyo, Japan Publications, 1985

COOKBOOKS

Aihara, Cornellia, *Macrobiotic Kitchen*, Tokyo, Japan Publications, 1983
Aihara, Cornellia, *The Do of Cooking*, Chico, CA, George Ohsawa Macrobiotic Foundation, 1972
Esko, Edward and Wendy, *Macrobiotic Cooking for Everyone*, Tokyo, Japan Publications, 1980
Esko, Wendy, *Introducing Macrobiotic Cooking*, Tokyo, Japan Publications, 1978
Estella, Mary, *Natural Foods Cookbook: Vegetarian Dairy-free Cuisine*, Tokyo, Japan Publications, 1985
Kushi, Aveline and Oredson, Olivia, *Macrobiotic Cooking for Cancer*, 1984.
Kushi, Aveline, *How to Cook with Miso*, Tokyo: Japan Publications, 1978
Kushi, Aveline with Alex Jack, *Aveline Kushi's Complete Guide to Macrobiotic Cooking for Health, Happiness and Peace*, Warner Publishing Co., 1984
Kushi, Aveline with Wendy Esko, *The Changing Seasons Macrobiotic Cookbook*, Wayne, NJ, Avery Publishing Group, 1984
Ohsawa, Lima, *Macrobiotic Cuisine*, Tokyo: Japan Publications, 1984

Other Macrotiotic or Related Books

Aihara, Herman, *Basic Macrobiotics* Tokyo, Japan Publications, 1985
Brown, Virginia with Susan Stayman, *Macrobiotic Miracle: How a Vermont Family Overcame Cancer*, Tokyo, Japan Publications, 1985
Dufty, William, *Sugar Blues*, New York, Warner, 1975
East West Journal (Periodical), Brookline, MA
Heidenry, Carolyn, *An Introduction to Macrobiotics: A Beginner's Guide to the Natural Way of Health*, Florence, Italy, Aladdin Press, 1984
Heidenry, Carolyn, *Making the Transition to a Macrobiotic Diet*, Florence, Italy, Aladdin Press, 1984
Heidenry, Carolyn, *Crossroads: America's Future—Decline or Ascent*, Florence Italy, Aladdin Press, 1984
Heidenry, Carolyn, *Yin Yang Coloring Book for Children*, Florence, Italy, Aladdin Press, 1984
Ineson, Rev. John, *The Way of Life: Macrobiotics and the Spirit of Christianity*, Tokyo, Japan Publications, 1985

Kohler, Jean and Mary Alice, *Healing Miracles from Macrobiotics*, West Nyack, NY, Parker, 1979

Kotzsch, Ronald E., Ph. D., *Macrobiotics: Yesterday and Today*, Tokyo, Japan Publications, 1985

Kushi, Aveline, *Lessons of Day and Night*, Wayne, NJ, Avery Publishing Group, 1984

Kushi, Aveline with Wendy Esko, *Growing Up Naturally: Macrobiotic Cooking for Healthy Children*, Tokyo, Japan Publications, 1985

Kushi, Aveline and Michio, *Macrobiotic Pregnancy and Care of the Newborn*, Tokyo, Japan Publications, 1984

Kushi, Aveline and Michio with Edward and Wendy Esko, *Macrobiotic Childcare and Family Health*, Tokyo, Japan Publications, 1985

Kushi, Michio, *The Book of Macrobiotics*, Tokyo, Japan Publications, 1977

Kushi, Michio, *Cancer and Heart Disease: The Macrobiotic Approach to Degenerative Disorders* (Revised edition), Tokyo, Japan Publications, 1985

Kushi, Michio, *Natural Healing Through Macrobiotics*, Tokyo, Japan Publications, 1978

Kushi, Michio, *The Era of Humanity*, Brookline, MA, East West Journal, 1980

Kushi, Michio, *How to See Your Health: The Book of Oriental Diagnosis*, Tokyo, Japan Publications, 1980

Kushi, Michio, *Your Face Never Lies*, Wayne, NJ, The Avery Publishing Group, 1983

Kushi, Michio, *The Book of Dō-In: Exercise for Physical and Spiritual Development*, Tokyo, Japan Publications, 1979

Kushi, Michio and the East West Foundation, *The Macrobiotic Approach to Cancer*, Wayne, NJ, The Avery Publishing Group, 1982

Kushi, Michio with Alex Jack, *The Cancer Prevention Diet*, NY, St. Martin's Press, 1983

Kushi, Michio with Alex Jack, *Eating to Your Heart's Content: The Natural Way to Relieve and Prevent Heart Attack, Stroke, and High Blood Pressure*, NY, St. Martin's Press, 1985

Kushi, Michio with Marc Van Cauwenberghe, *Macrobiotic Home Remedies*, Tokyo, Japan Publications, 1985

Mendelsohn, Robert, S., M.D., *Confessions of a Medical Heretic*, NY, Warner, 1979

Mendelsohn, Robert S., M.D., *Male Practice*, Chicago, Contemporary Books, 1980

Nussbaum, Elaine, *Recovery: From Cancer to Health Through Macrobiotics*, Tokyo, Japan Publications, 1985

Ohsawa, George, *Cancer and the Philosophy of the Far East*, Oroville, CA, George Ohsawa Macrobiotic Foundation, 1971

Ohsawa, George and Dufty, William, *You Are All Sanpaku*, NY, University Books, 1965

Sattilaro, Anthony, M.D. with Tom Monte, *Recalled by Life: The Story of My Recovery from Cancer*, Boston, Houghton-Mifflin, 1982

Tara, William, *Macrobiotics and Human Behavior*, Tokyo, Japan Publications, 1985

Index